D1359023

Anesthesiology

CLINICAL
DENTAL ANAESTHESIA

CLINICAL
DENTAL ANAESTHESIA
A MANUAL OF PRINCIPLES
AND PRACTICE

JAMES M. BELL

MB, BS, DA (Melbourne), FFARACS

Director of Anaesthesia, The Royal
Dental Hospital of Melbourne
Lecturer in Anaesthesia, School of
Dental Science, University of Melbourne
Honorary Anaesthetist, The Royal
Melbourne Hospital

BLACKWELL SCIENTIFIC PUBLICATIONS

OXFORD LONDON EDINBURGH MELBOURNE

© 1975 Blackwell Scientific Publications

Osney Mead, Oxford
85 Marylebone High Street, London W1M 3DE
9 Forrest Road, Edinburgh
P.O. Box 9, North Balwyn, Victoria, Australia

ISBN 0 632 00871 7

First published 1975

Distributed in the United States of America by
J.B.Lippincott Company, Philadelphia
and in Canada by
J.B.Lippincott Company of
Canada Ltd, Toronto

Printed in Great Britain by
Burgess & Son Ltd
Abingdon, Oxfordshire
and bound by
Kemp Hall Bindery
Osney Mead, Oxford

CONTENTS

PREFACE

What is dental sedation? Is it safe for dentists to use? Should dentists administer general anaesthesia, and should this be taught to dental undergraduates?

It is questions of this sort which specialist anaesthetists ask about clinical dental anaesthesia. If they read some of the available writings on the subject they will feel like intruders in a field where they are not wanted and seem almost to be scarcely needed.

The specialist anaesthetist has been accustomed to view dental anaesthesia from a distance, and to take the attitude that its problems can be easily solved. As he sees it, there is 'over-use' of general anaesthesia in the dental school. He knows that there are many dentists who manage all their patients with local, never needing to have recourse to general anaesthesia—his own dentist is probably just such a man! There will be the occasional case needing a general anaesthetic, of course, and there is oral surgery to be done—but these are dealt with as hospital in-patients.

The anaesthetist who is actively involved in dental school practice takes a different view: he would not remain there otherwise. He sees the simple efficacy of the classical methods which so nicely solve the problems with which the dentist is confronted. The techniques are satisfactory and safe in his hands; he can see no need for change.

These views are poles apart, and attempts to reconcile them have generally been fruitless. Too many specialist anaesthetists are openly critical of every feature of dental school practice—not only the over-use of anaesthesia, but the apparatus, the position, the dentist-anaesthetist—they can see nothing good in it. The dental school anaesthetist finds the ideas and methods of the specialist anaesthetist cumbersome and complex, and unrealistically restrictive in relation to the needs of the dental patient.

First-hand experience of general anaesthesia and sedation for dentistry convinced me that these needed urgently to be brought into the discipline of general anaesthesia. Specialist anaesthetists had to be attracted into the dental school; it was essential to modify the practice of dental anaesthesia to the point where it was acceptable to them.

The first half of this book is an account of this practice, its background and some justification for it. Its place in teaching is examined also, for this, and the related consideration of motivation, are of importance. Some dentists find working on nervous patients with unsupplemented local analgesia rather unpleasant; this is the principal factor which motivates them to give sedation and even general anaesthetics to their patients. Those who recommend that dental general anaesthetics be given only by trained anaesthetists overlook the point that specialists may be poorly motivated to do this kind of work.

The question of the training which a dentist should have to equip him to carry out sedation procedures safely is important. Suffice to say here that exposure, as an undergraduate, to an enlightened practice of anaesthesia is a good basis for postgraduate study.

ANAESTHETIC REGISTRAR TRAINING

When dental anaesthesia is properly established as part of the discipline of general anaesthesia, this problem tends to diminish. The anaesthetist in training expects to do his stint in anaesthesia for various special branches of surgery, and is keen to learn what he can from each one. Dentistry is now no exception, and is revealed as an unexcelled medium for teaching every aspect of airway care, in the lightly anaesthetized patient in particular. Senior anaesthetists of today who gained experience in this field by practical experience with such techniques as 'open drop ether' tend to decry the shortcomings of the younger anaesthetist in this regard. The modern anaesthetic registrar has difficulty in a general teaching hospital, in gaining practical experience in airway care under light anaesthesia—but participation in dental school practice will give him all of this and more. Opportunities abound for practical experience in almost every technical aspect of general anaesthesia in conditions of extreme safety. Dental anaesthesia is demonstrated here as a veritable 'paradigm of clinical anaesthesia'—if full advantage is taken of this aspect, then many problems of teaching disappear.

Some features of the text may require explanation. I have avoided giving detail in descriptions of technique, with few exceptions. Practice in general anaesthesia varies in detail from place to place. What is required is for the practice of general anaesthesia in a particular place to be thoroughly applied there to dental school anaesthesia. Such descriptions as are given of anaesthetic techniques contain enough detail for a specialist anaesthetist to comprehend and apply them. In the section on sedation (Part III), the objective has been to elucidate these techniques for the benefit, primarily, of the specialist anaesthetist. He needs to get into the dental school and learn at first hand to use these methods. Then perhaps they will receive a continual critical assessment and may be taught to dentists in a sounder manner than has sometimes been the case.

There are obvious omissions, of which two examples will be noted. No statistics are produced to justify methods described. An account is given of non-endotracheal methods (for convenience termed 'open') for use on out-patients: what of the follow-up? Realistic dental anaesthetists are unimpressed by small series of cases; what is needed is a follow-up which ensures that any serious complication will not be overlooked. Our association with the Royal Children's Hospital, Melbourne, and other teaching hospitals whose registrars attend our practice virtually ensures that we will hear of any serious complications. No case of post-anaesthetic pulmonary complication is known to have followed our non-endotracheal anaesthesia. One of our in-patients, however, did develop an acute aspiration pneumonia within 24 hours of an impeccably given endotracheal anaesthetic in the operating theatre.

No mention is made of some features dear to the hearts of dental anaesthetists. Cardiac arrhythmias are fascinating, but are too good an excuse for side-tracking. The current need is for anaesthetists to participate actively in dental school practice, not to fiddle with gadgets.

Mouth packing is an example of a fetish which obsesses some practical dental anaesthetists: more emphasis is put, quite deliberately, on active interference at need than on perfection in packing, for this is the lesson which is most needed now.

I shall be very disappointed with people who slavishly adopt the methods described. I should prefer them to argue and criticize, and would then feel that my labours have not been in vain.

ACKNOWLEDGEMENTS

Thanks are due to Professor Peter C. Reade, Chairman of the Department of Dental Medicine and Surgery, University of Melbourne, who provided the stimulus for writing this book and the facilities of his department for its preparation. In the clinical field my gratitude is expressed to Mr John Campbell, Senior Lecturer in Oral Surgery, University of Melbourne, and to Mr W.T. Smith, Dental Superintendent, The Royal Dental Hospital of Melbourne, who were chiefly responsible for educating me in the art of non-endotracheal anaesthesia for dentistry, and proved most adaptable in the face of the changes which were instituted. Mr John Godfrey of the Dental Staff of the Hospital co-operated in my early efforts at sedation and deserves thanks for his skill and patience.

The clinical illustrations are the work of Mr T. Dobrostanski of the University Department of Clinical Photography, whose co-operation has been unfailing. Acknowledgment is made of illustrations from other sources, Figure 1 is reproduced by courtesy of Messrs Churchill-Livingstone, and photographs for Figures 38, 39, 40, 41 and 43 were kindly provided by Medishield Division of CIG (The Commonwealth Industrial Gases Ltd, Australia).

The procedures described have been used and modified by many staff anaesthetists of the Royal Dental Hospital of Melbourne, to all of whom I express my gratitude.

I am grateful to Mr Peter Jones of Blackwell Scientific Publications (Australia) Pty Ltd, who has been a ready source of advice and assistance at all stages, and to the parent company at Oxford for the patience they have shown with a novice author and for their efficient production of this book.

PART I

THE PRESENT

Differences over dental anaesthesia constitute a widespread dilemma. Various aspects of the dispute are highlighted in various parts of the world but the disagreement is similar everywhere. The administration of general anaesthesia has traditionally been a right of the dentist—but it is a right which the modern anaesthetist questions. Modern anaesthesia as a whole, however, has tended to neglect the needs of dentistry—to be rather unhelpful—which forces the dental profession to provide for its own needs. The extent to which this is done in any place depends largely upon its traditions.

On the North American continent dental anaesthesia is very much in the hands of the dental profession, of oral surgeons in particular. Teaching in dental schools, of general anaesthesia and sedation is mainly carried out by dentists. Few anaesthesiologists take part. Those who do seem to act as mentors or advisers to individual teachers rather than exerting a general influence.

In the United Kingdom, dental schools usually have a specialist anaesthetist in charge of general anaesthesia and responsible for teaching, although much is still done by dentists. The majority of these dentists who are active in the field of sedation and anaesthesia appreciate the guidance of specialist anaesthetists and accept it readily. The dentist is at times critical, however, of the anaesthetic establishment for its apparent aloofness from the basic problems of dentistry.

The anaesthetist who is involved in dental school practice and teaching has sometimes been forced by circumstances, by pressure of work, patient numbers and the demands of undergraduate training to divest himself of much of his medicine and to become a mere instructor in a craft. It is for this reason that emphasis is placed here on the anaesthetist's role as physician and medical consultant. This is necessary to his adequate performance as an anaesthetist. If he is to be an effective ambassador for medicine it is vital.

In the field of dental sedation, problems can readily become blurred by disagreement over matters of detail. One has therefore tended to emphasize first the overriding need in the dental school for sound practice and teaching of general anaesthesia. With acceptance of this it may prove easier to extend the influence of anaesthetists into the newer field of sedation.

CHAPTER 1
ANAESTHETISTS AND DENTISTRY
THE PRESENT POSITION

In most dental schools, general anaesthesia is practised chiefly in relation to exodontia on out-patients. It is represented in teaching as a simple technical exercise. The dental undergraduate is provided with a lecture course on the physiology, pharmacology and practice of anaesthesia and is then taught to administer general anaesthesia.

In medical schools, general anaesthesia is an established postgraduate discipline. Such teaching as undergraduates receive is no longer directed chiefly towards imparting practical skill in the administration of anaesthesia. In so far as this is taught, it is with emphasis on teaching emergency resuscitation and airway care in the unconscious patient. A broader view is given of anaesthesia, so that the student may appreciate its potential and see the lessons of therapeutics and physiology which arise out of its practice. It is stressed that the anaesthetist is a physician: he has the personal responsibility of determining his patient's condition before the administration to assess fitness for the procedure intended. His findings here guide him in decisions relating to choice of anaesthetic technique and general management of the case. The modern specialist anaesthetist has an increasing involvement also in post-operative and intensive care.

In the circumstances in which the specialist anaesthetist makes contact with dental surgery, he is most likely dealing with cases for which in-patient endotracheal anaesthesia is appropriate. He may fail to realize that, for simple exodontia on healthy patients, another method—a different approach altogether—may not only be feasible, but in fact may be the technique of choice.

The practice of the dental school stands apart, and although many specialist anaesthetists see it in the light of a failure to develop as it should, through its remaining in isolation, those who participate find in it many excellent features. They are loath to allow any suggestion of a 'take over' by specialist anaesthetists: there is a feeling that this would mean an end to simplicity.

To the specialist anaesthetist, there are evident deficiencies in the dental school practice. Pre-anaesthetic medical assessment tends to be minimized as being largely unnecessary. The concept that the patient's medical condition may be a guide in the choice of anaesthetic is inapplicable because, as a rule, only one method is used—there is no choice. The anaesthetist is usually not a specialist; there may indeed be a dentist administering the anaesthetic. Yet dental anaesthesia over all has an excellent safety record, and many experienced anaesthetists find it satisfactory despite apparent contraventions of the principles which receive emphasis in the medical school. The reasons are not difficult to find.

The services of a skilled physician anaesthetist will most benefit the critically ill patient. Where such a patient is to undergo surgery of some magnitude there may be a need to use a complex anaesthetic technique, and to employ the methods of intensive care for the support of life for the period of surgery and beyond. In out-patient dental anaesthesia, the surgery is intrinsically free from serious morbidity and much care is taken to select healthy patients. In such circumstances the practice of simple methods is most appropriate—complexity is largely unnecessary. It is well to avoid, especially in out-patients, the potential for complications inherent in some of the procedures ordinarily used by the specialist anaesthetist for inpatients.

The administration of general anaesthesia by dentists may puzzle the young anaesthetist to whom general anaesthesia has always been a special branch of medicine. Consideration of the historical background helps to elucidate this point. The problems which faced the dentist of thirty to forty years ago in seeking painless extraction of teeth for his patients are most significant. Local analgesics of the day were either dangerous or ineffective by comparison with those of the present. Extraction was too often sought only when infection was well established. There were no antibiotics—the need for general anaesthesia was very great.

HISTORICAL OUTLINE

General anaesthesia for dentistry has been practised by dentists since its inception. It was originally used to induce unconsciousness briefly for extraction of teeth by simple inhalation with the patient sitting up in the dentist's chair—the usual position for dental treatment. This passed through many phases, initially it was inhalation of nitrous oxide pure or mixed with air, with inevitable hypoxia. Even after progression to use of nitrous oxide and oxygen mixtures it was still felt that the full effect of nitrous oxide could be obtained only when used in concentrations in excess of 80 per cent, which made restriction of the oxygen supply inevitable. The cyanosis which resulted was described in text books for many years as a clinical feature of nitrous oxide anaesthesia (Minnitt and Gillies 1948a), but it is only fair to mention that general anaesthesia administered by medical practitioners of that era for general surgery also involved hypoxia in many cases when nitrous oxide was used. Dentists usually confined their anaesthesia to brief administrations on healthy patients, and this brevity has been a major factor in the low mortality of dental anaesthesia. It did, however, put a premium on speed on the part of the dentist operating. It seems as if his involvement in the anaesthesia made the dentist accept as inevitable poor operating conditions and the need for hasty surgery.

The effect of development of general anaesthesia on other fields of surgery was very different. It was not usual in these for the surgeon to give the anaesthetic, this was done by the patient's own physician, or by a physician skilled in using the anaesthetics of the day. The surgeon felt free to criticize the anaesthesia, and constructive criticism was a stimulus to improvement of methods. In pre-anaesthetic days, stringent limitations on scope and duration of surgery were inevitable, it involved little more than amputations and drainage of pus. When anaesthesia was able to provide an unconscious, quiescent patient, and deliberate surgery became feasible, the scope of surgical procedures expanded dramatically and has continued to do so.

General anaesthesia became widely practised in teaching hospitals and medical undergraduates received instruction in its use. The emphasis was on agents and techniques providing anaesthesia with muscular relaxation suited to major surgery, speed of recovery was not significant—the methods were unsuitable for out-patient use. If nitrous oxide were used other than by an expert, the evanescence of its effect would be nullified by liberal supplements of ether.

Much greater expertise in the use of nitrous oxide was developed by dentists. From the early part of this century it was quite usual for dental schools to train their undergraduates in administration of general anaesthesia. The theoretical instruction was generally sound, by the standards of the day and practical application, the practice of the 'gas room', gave an excellent basis for safe administration of a brief general anaesthetic for exodontia.

The main anaesthetic agent was nitrous oxide. If this were used correctly the procedure was smooth and the recovery excellent. The medical man of this time was likely to be quite unable to give safely a brief general anaesthetic for an out-patient dental procedure. Those who gained proficiency in administration of 'dental gas' usually did so by receiving instruction from a dentist. The supremacy of dentists in this field is acknowledged in a text book of anaesthesia of that time with the advice to a medical practitioner that, for an out-patient dental case he 'must have something more appropriate to offer than open chloroform or ether' and that, if inexperienced in the use of gas and oxygen he should 'hand over the responsibility . . . rather than take part in a robot performance in which he holds the mask while the gases are turned on and off by the dentist'. (Minnitt and Gillies 1948b).

It is relevant to note that the most cogent criticism currently levelled by dentists at specialist medical anaesthetists concerns their frequent inability to give a simple general anaesthetic for a brief dental case.

That is how one sees the background to the tradition of administration of general anaesthesia by the dentist. Considerable success has attended the continuation of this practice in many centres chiefly because of strict adherence to simple techniques of general anaesthesia. By contrast, the specialist anaesthetist is sometimes too little aware of the virtues of simple methods. His teaching hospital training in modern anaesthetic technology may give him a limited outlook. He knows, for example, that the use of neuromuscular blocking agents allows great facility in endotracheal intubation at the hands of an expert, and feels therefore that this must be the anaesthetic method of choice for all dental surgery. There is a widespread refusal on the part of specialist anaesthetists to countenance simple non-endotracheal anaesthesia for dental surgery. This, coupled with the dentists' unwillingness to accept the fact that endotracheal methods are needed in the dental school clinic constitutes the major point of contention. Critical examination of dental school practice of general anaesthesia must of course go beyond mere matters of technique, yet its pragmatic efficiency is not a sufficient basis on which to extol the practice. It is important in dental undergraduate teaching. When one asks whether or not it is fulfilling its teaching function however, the answer must depend on what one expects of it.

GENERAL ANAESTHETIC TEACHING

The dental undergraduate who knows as 'general anaesthesia' only the nasal administration of nitrous oxide to the seated patient can gain only a limited, inadequate view of anaesthesia. The fact that he may witness other forms of anaesthesia in other places perhaps heightens the bad educational effect of the practice of the 'gas room'. The most serious anachronism of this (which receives close attention in Chapter 3) is the organization which deprives the anaesthetist of the prerogative of making decisions, on the basis of the condition of the patient, about the type of anaesthetic to be used.

The dentist of the future may seldom undertake routine administration of general anaesthesia. He is, however, likely to employ sedation (see Part III Chapter 7). To do this safely it is essential that he have a broad, sound education in anaesthesia. The drugs and agents used for sedation are those of general anaesthesia. The mere definition of sedation as a state in which consciousness is retained will not ensure that patients do not become unconscious. The dentist who is to administer sedation safely must know thoroughly both the drugs that he uses and the state of his patient. He will require a high degree of technical skill in the means of airway maintenance and resuscitation in all circumstances. He must, in short, learn a great deal about the techniques of general anaesthesia, as well as gaining a sound understanding of the discipline.

Inadequacies of general anaesthetic teaching in the dental school militate against establishment of a good practice of sedation. 'Post graduate' courses in sedation will be of doubtful value unless there is a sound basic teaching for undergraduates. As to whether graduate dentists should practise sedation, it is stated that the decision to do this or not is for the dentist to take (Australian Dental Association 1971). This advice is sound, however, only if the dentist has been given an education in general anaesthesia which will provide him with an adequate basis for the decision.

Traditional anaesthetic methods do not give a good basis for teaching of sedation, nor should sedation be represented as a simple practical exercise. The undergraduate should be introduced early to a practice of anaesthesia as close as possible to ideal. One must aim high in this regard, and deliberately ignore considerations of expediency which have for so long perpetuated archaic practice.

PART II

GENERAL ANAESTHESIA

In this Part, an attempt is made to delineate a sound basis for application of the skills of the modern anaesthetist to the out-patient practice of dental anaesthesia. The practice and organization which is described and illustrated is that of the Royal Dental Hospital in Melbourne. To assist in the understanding of the clinical concepts set out, a brief description is given here of some features of this hospital with which one has the privilege of being associated.

There is a short stay ward in the hospital staffed by general trained nurses which provides inpatient care. Patients admitted to this are under the care of the Hospital dental staff. The accommodation available is small relative to the number of operations performed with general anaesthesia, there is still need for much to be done on an out-patient basis. The fact of having a ward bed readily available, however, encourages a high degree of freedom in the choice of out-patient methods and patient selection. The anaesthetist is less inhibited by consideration of the remote possibility of unforeseen difficulty or slow recovery if there is immediately available a ward bed to which he has some right, as distinct from the situation which exists in so many Dental Schools in which a delayed recovery in an out-patient means going 'cap in hand to beg a bed', which must tend to restrict the scope of out-patient general anaesthesia. This should be borne in mind if at times suggestions about out-patient management seem to be unduly facile.

Availability of in-patient facilities necessitates the making of decisions about the need for in-patient care in various cases. No longer is this facility so difficult of attainment that only extreme indications warrant its use. With the opportunity for close follow up of patients undergoing general anaesthesia, it becomes clear that the sequelae of endotracheal intubation per se in adults and older children are negligible: they constitute no more than a temporary minor inconvenience. Surgical complications are of greater significance—the most important being haemorrhage. This is the major reason for the emphasis which is placed on the fact that indications for in-patient treatment after general anaesthesia are to be sought more in the health of the patient, and in the nature of the surgery, than in the particular method of anaesthesia used.

CHAPTER 2
ENDOTRACHEAL ANAESTHESIA

Few advances have done more to increase the safety and scope of general anaesthesia than endotracheal intubation. The use of this technique has increased in company with other developments—in particular the safe use of neuromuscular blocking agents and the use of intermittent positive pressure respiration. The potential for providing a safe and certain airway with complete protection against soiling of the tracheo-bronchial passages makes endotracheal intubation a uniquely valuable technique in both general anaesthesia and resuscitation. It is the method of choice for major dental procedures, it is used by the specialist anaesthetist for oral surgery when the patient is in hospital. Yet there is still, as noted in Chapter 1 a body of opinion which holds that endotracheal intubation is by no means always indicated in general anaesthesia for dental surgery. An account is now given of the development of endotracheal anaesthesia with a consideration of its problems and complications, in an effort to establish what should be its place in dentistry.

CLINICAL DEVELOPMENT

This has occurred in three stages, the first technique being in clinical use from about the year 1912 onwards. It was the insufflation of anaesthetic vapour, ether or chloroform as a rule through a small bore catheter placed in the trachea with its end near the carina. Although this arrangement did not provide an artificial airway for the patient, it prevented obstruction due to laryngospasm, and adequate delivery of air and anaesthetic to the patient was assured. It provided a safe means of maintaining anaesthesia during surgery of the head and neck. The tube was introduced under deep inhalation anaesthesia using either digital manipulation or direct laryngoscopy, and a pharyngeal pack was carefully placed so that, while preventing soiling of the air passages it would still allow free expiration. This method had a long total span of use, because it became popular with otolaryngologists, if the anaesthetist was not skilled in laryngoscopy, the surgeon would place the catheter. The second stage was the development of the wide bore tube by Magill, after whom it is named, who was anaesthetist in the faciomaxillary unit at Sidcup, U.K., during and after the War of 1914–1918. The tubes which he used were much the same as those in use today. They were made of mineralized rubber and were generally passed blindly into the trachea by the nasal route. The most important feature of this development is that the wide bore tube ensured a free airway in almost any circumstances, offering, with a high degree of certainty, continuity and safety of anaesthesia, as well as allowing effective pharyngeal packing to prevent aspiration of foreign material.

The major disadvantage of these techniques until recent years was the deep inhalational anaesthesia needed for insertion of the tube. For major faciomaxillary surgery in particular, this limitation was accepted because it made possible the deliberate performance of precise surgery. Advances in surgery of cleft lip and palate, and of plastic repair to the face in general were due at least in part to the good conditions provided by the anaesthetist. Plastic surgery was second only to thoracic surgery as a stimulus to continual improvement of anaesthetic methods.

For dental extractions, although the idea of an assured airway may have been attractive, the technique was too formidable for routine use, and quite out of the question for out-patients. When endotracheal anaesthesia was at this stage of development, the open administration of 'nasal gas' was in many ways a far superior anaesthetic technique for performance of brief extraction of teeth. It is the third stage, the modern practice of using neuromuscular blocking agents to facilitate intubation which has removed the need for a deep plane of general anaesthesia—and has made feasible the employment of endotracheal anaesthesia on adults who are out-patients. This technique is familiar to specialist anaesthetists and will not be described in detail: the points which will receive attention are those relevant to its use in dental surgery. These are the means of avoidance of soiling of the air passages at all stages of the anaesthetic when surgery is performed in the mouth, nasotracheal intubation, and the use and limitations of the technique for children and for out-patients.

NASAL INTUBATION

An endotracheal tube may be introduced through the mouth or nose. When endotracheal anaesthesia routinely employed inhalation agents, a number of skilled anaesthetists used blind nasal intubation because in their hands it required a less deep plane of anaesthesia than that needed for direct laryngoscopy. The oral route is now more generally used in any case in which there is no special indication for the nasal route. The ease of direct laryngoscopy under anaesthesia with neuromuscular blockade is such that the direct approach is quite feasible. Although nasal intubation has inherent drawbacks, it is highly favoured for dentistry. There are the obvious advantages— that the mouth is left free, providing good access for surgery, and that intra-oral manipulations are less likely to dislodge or kink the tube. Further advantages of the nasal route concern facility of management of extubation. This should be effected when anaesthesia is very light and neuromuscular blockade is at least on the way to reversal, as a safeguard against aspiration of blood and débris. A problem which is likely to occur with an oral tube at this stage is that the lightly anaesthetized patient may bite on the tube which is still in place, causing respiratory obstruction, the correction of which is difficult. There is also the risk that the tube will become kinked or prematurely displaced during efforts to clear the mouth prior to extubation. Problems of this sort are largely avoided by use of a nasal tube. The tube will be well tolerated at a light plane of anaesthesia, and cannot be obstructed by biting. Suction to clear the mouth, and placement of packs to minimize bleeding can be deliberately carried out.

The technical problems of nasal endotracheal intubation are familiar, the indications for its use are almost never absolute. The anaesthetist needs to be able to weigh up its advantages and disadvantages. Introduction of the nasal tube is usually not difficult, but occasionally presents problems in cases where orotracheal intubation presents none. The lengths to which an anaesthetist should go to achieve nasotracheal intubation in any particular case will be a matter for judgment, based on the condition of the patient and the nature of the surgery, and a decision may be made in consultation with the surgeon. In cases where a nasal tube is particularly desired, but difficulty is encountered in passage of the tube through the nose to the pharynx, the following may be of use.

In case of difficulty the tendency to try immediately a tube of smaller diameter should be resisted. The smaller tube tends to wander into 'blind passages', a tube of appropriate size for the larynx can usually be made to traverse the nose. It is important to avoid the upper nasal cavity, one should tilt up the nasal tip and insert the well lubricated tube along the floor of the nose following the line of the roof of the mouth. If the passage of the tube is obstructed with the tip just short of the edge of the soft palate—this will usually be due to its impinging on lymphoid tissue in the lateral wall of the nasopharynx— it may be freed by a well lubricated index finger introduced through the mouth and passed up behind the soft palate. With the finger-nail on the posterior pharyngeal wall the finger is moved laterally so that the pulp slips behind the tube, which can then be hooked away from the lateral wall, and, with a push from without, advanced into the pharynx. It will be necessary to do this only if it has not been possible to pass the obstruction by rotating the external part of the tube to deviate its tip. This is more difficult in the case of most cuffed tubes because of the ridge formed by the pilot tube which limits rotation of the tube in the nasal cavity.

Blind nasal intubation

This can be learned only by practice—the guiding principles are simple. Current practice is to perform it on a patient who is anaesthetized, relaxed and apnoeic, and has been well oxygenated. A plain tube is easier to guide than a cuffed for the reason just mentioned. The patient is positioned with only slight flexion of the neck and with the head less extended than is usual for laryngoscopy. The tube is introduced and guided with the right hand while the left pushes the larynx posteriorly, virtually occluding the oesophagus, and finger and thumb on each side feel for the tip of the tube to the right or left of the larynx, the tube is withdrawn a little and redirected as needed. If it runs into the vallecula, more head flexion is required. Blind intubation, if easily achieved, is a delightful procedure. If it is difficult, ready resort should be had to laryngoscopy: the occasional hazards of profuse haemorrhage, displacement of a nasal polyp, or of the tube going astray in the submucosal plane are too unpleasant to risk overlooking.

Nasal intubation under vision is preferred—a laryngoscope should be inserted and the pharynx viewed even before introduction of the tube into the nostril. Nasal haemorrhage may be started by the very first contact of the tube with mucosa, and if not immediately recognized may quickly fill the pharynx with blood with a serious risk of aspiration into the trachea.

As most endotracheal tubes are made with bevel to the left, the right nostril is favoured unless obviously obstructed (Fig. 1), this is less important if a tube with a 'Murphy tip' is used (Fig. 2). When the end of the tube is lying in the pharynx it is picked up with the Magill forceps and placed in the larynx, an assistant being directed to push

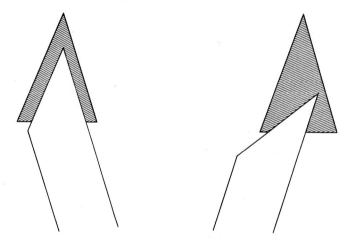

Fig. 1.   The bevel on an endotracheal tube is so placed as to make it easier to insert from the right side.

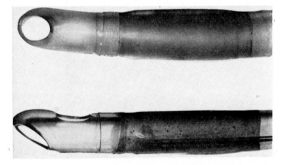

Fig. 2.   This pattern of tip makes passage of the endotracheal tube easier and less traumatic both to nasal cavity and to larynx.

the tube into the nose as needed. Because of the usual posture of the patient for laryngoscopy, with neck flexed and head extended, the tip of the tube tends to impinge on the anterior wall of the larynx or trachea, and this may impede its passage. This tendency is overcome by application of some or all of the following:

1. The tip of the tube is placed well posteriorly in the larynx and gently held back with forceps while it is pushed between the vocal cords—the tube is grasped at least 2–3 cm from its tip for this purpose (Fig. 3).

2. As the tip is advanced between the cords, the end of the laryngoscope in the vallecula is allowed to drop posteriorly a little (Fig. 4). This brings the larynx and trachea more into line with the tube, the posterior portion of the glottis should be kept in view to ensure that the tube does not slip unnoticed into the oesophagus.

3. If this is not successful the pressure on the laryngoscope is relaxed completely and the head is flexed. While a gentle attempt is made to advance the tube with the right hand, the left manipulates the larynx backwards and from side to side (Fig. 5). The tube will usually slip into the trachea but an immediate check

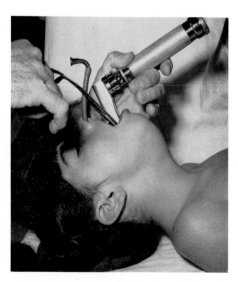

Fig. 3. Elevation of the laryngeal aperture by the beak of the laryngoscope accentuates the tendency of the tube to impinge on the anterior wall of the larynx.

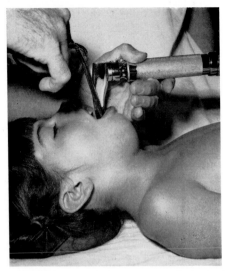

Fig. 4. Dropping the beak of the laryngoscope allows the larynx to fall posteriorly and facilitates insertion of the tube with the aid of Magill forceps.

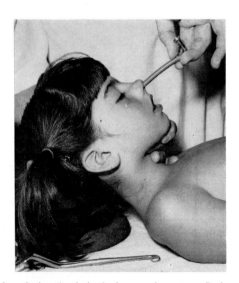

Fig. 5. After placing the tip in the laryngeal aperture, flexion of the head and manipulation of the larynx may achieve passage of the tube into the trachea.

should be made—by listening at the tube while sharp pressure is made on the chest—to ensure that the tube has entered the trachea and not the oesophagus.

Selection of endotracheal tubes

Rubber is a reliable material for endotracheal tubes, especially for brief procedures. A rubber cuff tends to undergo more even inflation and perhaps provides more even pressure over its length than is the case with some plastic cuffs. Plastic tubes have some advantages over rubber which are mostly of significance in long cases. Difficulty of sterilization, and liability of failure of cuffs are practical problems in the use of some plastic tubes. Thickness of wall, being sometimes greater in plastic than in rubber tubes, is most significant in small size tubes.

Diameter of tube

A preliminary decision about size of endotracheal tube is made on the basis of age, sex and size of patient, and an estimate of the size of the larynx, which may be made in various ways. Palpation of the larynx—of the cricoid ring in particular—is of value in adults. In boys about puberty note should be taken of the depth of voice: if the voice has 'broken', a larger size tube will be needed. A tube of 8 mm internal diameter is the largest usually passed nasally and is suitable for most adults. When an endotracheal tube is passed through the mouth it is easy to determine if the size is correct by whether it is a tight or loose fit in the larynx and trachea. When the nasal route is used however, the firmness of the fit in the nasal cavity may prevent recognition of the fact that the tube is an unduly tight fit in the trachea. This will rarely be of significance in adults but in children is most important; pressure on the mucosa of the subglottic region by an unduly large endotracheal tube is a major precipitating cause of post-anaesthetic stridor. In a small child the mucosal swelling resulting from such pressure may lead to a serious degree of respiratory obstruction. It is wise, in children, to try a tube for size by inserting it through the mouth into the trachea before passing it nasally. In this way a tight fitting tube may be readily detected and a smaller one substituted.

Length of nasal tubes

There is a close correlation between internal diameter and appropriate length of nasal endotracheal tubes. If tubes are cut to the standard lengths indicated in Table 2.1 it will be rare for the tube to be long enough to reach the lower end of the trachea, but the tip will be well below the glottis. Departures from this are most likely to occur in small children, with tubes from 4 to 5 mm diameter. A careful check of ventilation of both lungs should always be made after fully inserting the endotracheal tube to detect accidental entry of the tube into one bronchus. The greater length noted for cuffed tubes is to ensure that the top of the cuff rests below the larynx: that the cuff is entirely within the trachea.

Table 2.1. Nasal endotracheal tubes
Internal diameter related to age of patient and to appropriate length of tube and correct size of connection. (Magill 'Nasal' Elbow.)

	Diameter (millimetres)	Length (centimetres)	Age of patient (years)	Magill Elbow (number)
Cuffed tubes	8·0	28	15 Adult	12
	7·5	27	13–14	11
	7·0	26	11–12	10
	6·5	24	9–10	10
	6·0	23	7–8	9
Uncuffed (plain) tubes	6·5	22	9–10	10
	6·0	21	7–8	9
	5·5	20	5–6	8
	5·0	19	3–4	8
	4·5	18	2	7
	4·0	17	Under 2	7

MUSCLE RELAXANT DRUGS

Endotracheal intubation is carried out with the aid of a neuromuscular blocking agent, and brief consideration will now be given to the selection of the appropriate muscle relaxant. Anaesthetists who have a limited acquaintance with dental surgery tend to use a short acting relaxant of the 'depolarizing' type—suxamethonium. They feel relaxation is needed only for intubation and that anaesthesia can be maintained by inhalation; this policy is not always sound. Quick achievement of full recovery from general anaesthesia is desirable in dental cases because there may be post-operative bleeding—the cough reflex should be active at an early stage of recovery. This may be delayed if inhalation anaesthesia with a potent supplement has been prolonged.

If a procedure is expected to take more than perhaps fifteen minutes, the use of a longer acting 'non-depolarizing' muscle relaxant, d-tubocurarine or gallamine, may be desirable. If the operation is on the posterior part of the mouth this applies more strongly, it is easier to retract the tongue in a patient who is well relaxed. With careful dosage, based primarily on body weight, making allowance for obesity or youth as indicated by experience, the use of these drugs, even on out-patients can be quite satisfactory. An anticholinesterase-neostigmine with atropine is given at the conclusion to reverse residual effects, and the patient observed for sufficient time to ensure that reversal is complete. The recognition of signs suggestive of residual neuromuscular blockade such as restlessness in children, staring of the eyes and muscular twitching in adults, during recovery from the effects of anaesthesia is of importance when curare type drugs are used.

The advantages of using curare type muscle relaxant drugs in dental cases go beyond these, however. If teaching of anaesthetic registrars is undertaken in the dental clinic, there is much to be said for discouraging the use of suxamethonium, except for cases in which there is a positive indication for its use. These indications are familiar, the patient who may have a full stomach is one, or the patient in whom not only is a difficulty anticipated with intubation, but in whom there may also be some problem in ventilating the lungs by other means. Those who wish to learn thoroughly the art of tracheal intubation are advised against the routine use of suxamethonium. It makes many intubations very easy, but its short duration of action allows little time for development of a deliberate technique, and for gaining familiarity with landmarks, which is so essential to achievement of any difficult intubation. When difficulty arises, moreover, one is forced to use repeated doses of suxamethonium—which may not be desirable—or else the instructor must take over and insert the tube.

If the dosage and timing is appropriate, and the patient presents no problem in ventilation of the lungs using a face mask, the use of a non-depolarizing relaxant can be most valuable in teaching endotracheal intubation. After oxygenation is effected, the registrar can introduce the laryngoscope with a quite unhurried deliberation. The anatomy can be seen and carefully studied, the effect of raising the head to flex the neck and improve access to the glottis can be plainly demonstrated. If intubation is not achieved soon enough, one can desist, ventilate the patient, give an increment of intravenous anaesthetic if needed, and then repeat the attempt. Two or three cases attempted in this manner can give the anaesthetist a greater depth of experience than would be gleaned from many more quick intubations using suxamethonium. A further advantage of the use of a non-depolarizing relaxant is that the residual muscle tone and slight movement which is usual forms a sound introduction to the acquisition of the more difficult, but very important skill of laryngoscopy on the lightly anaesthetized patient. In the practice of non-endotracheal anaesthesia in the Dental Clinic, there are many opportunities to learn and practise this important technique.

THROAT PACKING

This is an important factor in protection of the air passages against ingress of foreign material—it is necessary that its purpose be understood and the packing correctly carried out. The use of a cuffed endotracheal tube does not render the use of a throat pack unnecessary—nor is the use of a throat pack with a cuffed tube merely a case of double protection: the two things serve different functions. The cuff on the tube, if correctly inflated, prevents material from passing the cuff into the distal part of the trachea and into the bronchi while the tube is in place. The cuff will protect against inhalation of regurgitated gastric contents, a pack alone will not protect against this. If there is to be haemorrhage into the mouth with the risk of blood or foreign matter entering the pharynx, use of a pack is mandatory. If blood is allowed free ingress to the pharynx, and clots there, laryngoscopy prior to extubation will reveal blood clot in every part of the pharynx—complete removal of this by suction before extubation is difficult and may be traumatic.

The important function of a pharyngeal pack is to occupy space in the pharynx so that blood will not form clots there. If it is thought of as a 'plug in a hole', the tendency will be to pack too tightly, with a risk of damage to fauces, soft palate and uvula, or of compression or kinking of the endotracheal tube. The pack should not be inserted dry, it should be soaked in water, normal saline, or paraffin oil, all excess should be removed before insertion of the pack. Most important in avoiding trauma are gentle placement, avoiding compression of soft tissue, and the quality of the gauze itself. Packing gauzes vary in quality, some being extremely 'rough'. A practical demonstration of the quality of a gauze is provided for the anaesthetist by using a portion of gauze pack as he would a handkerchief, to wipe his nose: he will learn at first hand how traumatic some types of gauze can be to a mucosal surface!

The retained pharyngeal pack

Whenever a pharyngeal pack is used, there is a risk that it will be left in place when the endotracheal tube is removed, and endanger the life of the patient by asphyxiation. This risk is inherent in the use of a throat pack, it is accepted because the use of the pack minimizes another hazard—the risk of inhalation of blood clot during recovery.

It is doubtful if there is any certain method of avoiding the hazard of leaving behind the throat pack on extubation. It is wise to employ routinely several safeguards, and to rely implicitly on none. If everyone with responsibility for care of the unconscious patient is keenly 'airway conscious', and anaesthetist and surgeon investigate the mouth and pharynx on any suggestion of airway difficulty which is not fully relieved by simple measures, the retained pack will not be overlooked. All gauzes used in the mouth in oral surgery should be 'checked in and out' in accordance with standard theatre procedure, and the throat pack should be included in this count. In operating theatres used mostly for general surgery, the throat pack may be overlooked by the theatre nursing staff despite obsequiously careful checking of all other gauzes. Mechanical precautions such as leaving an end of the pack out of the mouth or attaching a string which hangs out have high nuisance value to the surgeon and have been seen to fail. Laryngoscopy and pharyngeal toilet by the anaesthetist before extubation is good practice—but it is still possible for a pack to be overlooked, especially if it is a rather small one for the patient's size and is soaked with blood.

Inclusion of a radio-opaque marker in the gauze of the throat pack suggests a detachment from clinical reality. In contrast with the case of a pack accidentally sewn up in a belly, where radiographic location should precede deliberate removal, suspicion of a retained throat pack should lead to immediate definitive steps towards freeing of airway: there is no place here for radiography. A further point is that the radio-opaque thread is often rough and more traumatic to tissues than the gauze pack.

The problem of retained throat pack is likely to arise when some circumstance is unusual, as it is important for the anaesthetist to be alerted by such an occurrence, two examples are mentioned. In a case of multistage facial restoration by a plastic surgeon the anaesthetist anticipated that the attachment of the tubed pedicle would involve the cheek and the angle of the mouth, and inserted a throat pack. The mouth was not in fact involved, the anaesthetist was misled by the absence of soiling of the mouth, and distracted, and discouraged from laryngoscopy by the need to retain the position of the arm to which the pedicle was attached. He removed the tube with the pack still in place. It was the occurrence of respiratory difficulty some time after extubation which led the house-surgeon to put a finger into the mouth and pharynx, and to find and remove the pack.

On another occasion a delay in return of spontaneous respiration at the end of a procedure which did not involve the mouth, contrary to what had been anticipated, led to the patient being transferred to the recovery room with tube and pack still in place. Before extubation some two hours later, the anaesthetist performed routine laryngo-scopy, and was most surprised to see the throat pack, the insertion of which had been forgotten. The occurrence of any departure from routine alerts the experienced clinician to take extra care in every aspect of management of the case.

EXTUBATION

This is of importance in that it marks the termination of airway protection afforded by the endotracheal tube and the resumption of dynamic protection by the return of the patient's own protective reflexes. It is an area where principles can readily be enunciated, but it can be learned only by experience. In theory, the endotracheal tube will be tolerated only while protective reflexes are completely in abeyance, yet it is important that reflex activity must return imme-diately the tube is removed if the patient is to be safe. In practice reliance is placed on the phenomenon of adaptation: after the larynx and trachea are able to react to the tube its presence will be tolerated if it is not moved to stimulate new areas of sensitive mucosa. This is why removal of the endotracheal tube so often is followed immediately by a vigorous cough. One does not place implicit reliance on the occurrence and efficacy of this return of reflex activity, especially in the case with actual or potential bleeding in the mouth. It is wise to turn the patient on his side before extubation—it is often convenient to move him from operating table to trolley in the process of turning. With the patient in the lateral position and slightly head down, pharyngeal aspiration is completed, the cuff deflated and the endotracheal tube removed from the larynx. A further aspiration of the pharynx may be performed by placing the sucker nozzle on the end of the tube, once the tip is clear of the larynx. This ensures that the nasopharynx is free from mucus and blood clot which could be inhaled. The head is extended, and a pharyngeal airway inserted if indicated: a face mask replaces the endotracheal adapter and gentle inflation with oxygen is intermittently effected. Laryngospasm, although rarely serious, is an ever present hazard following extubation, and the cardinal rules for preventing this inco-ordinate overaction of the glottic reflex are:

1. Keep foreign material from the region of the larynx—by posture and suction.

2. Administer oxygen with gentle intermittent positive pressure—so that minor inco-ordination of the glottis will not be aggravated by hypoxia, and because gentle, rhythmic inflation is a potent aid to re-establishment of respiration.

These measures are especially important in cases where the action of a curare type neuromuscular blocking agent has just been reversed by administration of neostigmine: it is important to maintain ventilation while an assessment is made of the completeness of the reversal. Important criteria of this are ability to give a sharp cough, to swallow, to take a deep breath with expansion of the thorax and no tracheal tug. It is important to recognize that early post-anaesthetic laryngeal stridor may be due to residual neuromuscular blockade: in this case there is usually diminished respiratory drive, and laryngoscopy shows rather floppy vocal cords which do not abduct fully. A further dose of neostigmine with atropine will dramatically cure the condition, as a rule, but oxygenation should be continued meanwhile.

Difficulty may be encountered at this stage in the patient who has had a full clearance of teeth, and is left with upper and lower alveolar ridges, commonly still bleeding a little, which tend to make close contact and obstruct the oral airway during recovery. If a nasal endotracheal tube has just been removed, and there is a poor nasal airway associated with epistaxis the problem is further aggravated. The presence of blood in the mouth makes the 'head low' position desirable—this tends to increase haemorrhage. Inspiration past narrowly separated bleeding gums may result in aspiration of blood. If anaesthesia is deep, this is dangerous: if light, it results in coughing and laryngospasm, and the respiratory efforts which follow increase venous pressure which further aggravates the haemorrhage. This type of unpleasant vicious circle during recovery from anaesthesia is not of course confined to dental surgery. It is one with which the anaesthetist learns to cope, and the proper practice of general anaesthesia for dental surgery offers, perhaps, the safest environment in which to learn to deal with it. Better to gain experience in management of this technical problem on a healthy patient in good condition than to try to cope with it for the first time on an accident case perhaps with complicating factors such as multiple injuries and advanced surgical shock.

The handling of the problem is learnt as a practical exercise, a few points are mentioned which may be of value. Bleeding will be minimal at the hands of a surgeon who works skilfully, sutures effectively, and packs each section or quadrant after completion. If working with an unfamiliar surgeon the anaesthetist is well advised to examine the mouth before lightening anaesthesia or reversing neuromuscular blockade: if there is bleeding, it should be dealt with deliberately—whether by pressure, suture or other means—before extubation. A useful measure is to insert a large (6 cm × 12 cm) gauze covered pack between the jaws on each side, with a Guedel airway between the packs if needed. Careful avoidance of airway obstruction is the other important factor—this advice should be effectively conveyed to recovery staff.

AFTER CARE

The anaesthetist needs to take an interest in the recovery of his patients from general anaesthesia. Complications which arise in recovery are complications of the anaesthetic: it is of little use to avoid intra-operative airway obstruction or soiling if the means of doing this causes later problems to an undue extent. Where a patient has been subjected to neuromuscular blockade and endotracheal intubation, close observation by a skilled person is mandatory during recovery. The patient is held in a recovery area which is desirably adjacent to the theatre, until he is conscious and his vital reflexes are functioning normally. During this time he should be on a trolley in the lateral position, supervised by a trained nurse with sucker and oxygen to hand. Pulse and blood pressure are observed and coughing, haemorrhage, vomiting and return of consciousness are noted. The nurse in attendance needs to be skilled in management of the airway, pharyngeal aspiration and capable of intermittent positive pressure breathing if needed. She should be keenly aware of the indications for seeking the help of the anaesthetist, some further details of this are dealt with in Chapter 6 (page 85).

After effects

It is usual for a patient to suffer some discomfort following endo-tracheal intubation: it is unusual for this to be serious in adults. Hoarseness and sore throat are common, they are not as a rule severe and are mainly of short duration. Their occurrence may sometimes be foreseen, being related to particular technical difficulties such as attempting intubation with inadequate relaxation.

In children the sequelae of intubation may be more serious, the risk of precipitating sub-glottic oedema by use of too large a tube has been noted. The possible occurrence of post-operative stridor from this cause is the main factor which limits the use of endotracheal anaesthesia in children as out-patients—it is important to appreciate its incidence relative to age of patient. Stridor from sub-glottic oedema is most serious under three years of age. In the post-operative period, these children may rapidly progress from slight croup to severe respiratory difficulty. Endotracheal anaesthesia on children as young as this should preferably be undertaken only by a skilled paediatric anaesthetist or in a well equipped hospital. In children of average size it is not a serious problem over six years of age. The use of endotracheal anaesthesia for extraction of permanent molars in the older child, therefore, is quite safely undertaken on an out-patient basis. Detailed indications for endotracheal intubation in dental surgery will not be considered at this stage: a knowledge of feasible alternatives is essential for this. The matter will be considered after non-endotracheal methods have been fully examined.

CHAPTER 3
NON-ENDOTRACHEAL TECHNIQUE

The outstanding feature which the specialist anaesthetist sees in dental out-patient general anaesthesia is that a non-endotracheal technique of anaesthesia is used for extraction of teeth. He is accustomed to using endotracheal anaesthesia for dental extractions, and can satisfy himself that this is justifiable. He is generally unaware of any justification for the administration of dental anaesthetics without intubation, apart from the pragmatic ones of long usage and statistically low morbidity and mortality.

A complete consideration of out-patient dental anaesthesia should deal with the justification of methods other than endotracheal intubation and should examine both theoretical and practical aspects of a variety of techniques. In this chapter an account will be given of a modified practice of out-patient dental anaesthesia which has been developed over the last five years at the Royal Dental Hospital of Melbourne by specialist anaesthetists. This practice evolved from application of the best precepts and practice of modern anaesthesia to the problems of dental extractions—and by taking cognizance of older methods. To describe new techniques *de novo* would be unfair— it would fail to acknowledge a debt not only to older methods, but also to the expertise of dental colleagues, whose skill and experience with non-endotracheal techniques have been indispensable in development of modified methods. This chapter will therefore begin with a description of a classical technique of nasal administration of nitrous oxide—choosing a fairly typical procedure such as is still currently practised in many dental schools—and a careful appraisal of its shortcomings.

CLASSICAL NASAL GAS

The patient is seated upright in a dental chair, which is usually tilted slightly to a reclining position for greater stability and ease of access.

Induction of anaesthesia may be by intravenous injection, the main anaesthetic is nitrous oxide and oxygen, commonly supplemented with halothane and administered by a nasal mask (Fig. 6). When a sufficient depth of anaesthesia is attained the mouth is held open with a gag or prop, and extractions are performed, mouth packs being

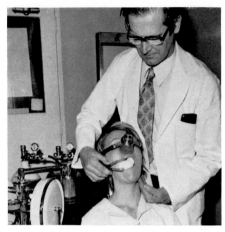

Fig. 6. Shows some important features of the 'Classical Nasal Gas' administration.

placed to protect the airway and the jaw supported to maintain free breathing. The anaesthetic is lightened as the operation proceeds and is withdrawn towards its conclusion: the patient, with packs over his tooth sockets is leant forward ready to expectorate in a dish. He is moved to a recovery area by walking assisted, by wheelchair, or by carrying in the case of children. In reasonably expert hands—and it must be recognized that anaesthetist and dentist form a team—this procedure appears expeditious and safe: it has an extremely low mortality. It has been associated however with features which are viewed with disfavour by modern eyes and these will now be examined.

Hypoxia and positive pressure

The use of the 'Demand Flow' apparatus of the McKesson type (Fig. 7) which is still widely practised in dentistry is closely related to the former practice of deliberate use of hypoxia in anaesthesia and of continuous positive pressure, and these will therefore be considered

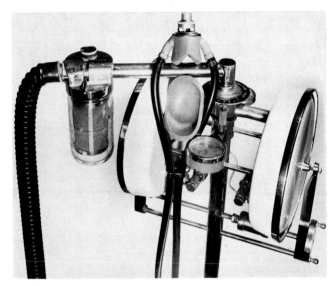

Fig. 7.   A demand flow machine of the 'McKesson' type. The vaporizer was generally used for Trichlorethylene, the single lever on a graduated scale controlled the oxygen percentage.

together. The circumstances in which hypoxic induction was used and the reasons for its popularity need to be understood. There were no intravenous anaesthetics and the available volatile supplement was ether. The problem was to subdue briefly a robust patient for extraction of a small number of teeth, and to have him ready to resume activity within a short space of time: for this the method was efficacious. The Demand Flow apparatus was vital to success; only with its high flow rates to meet peak inspiratory demand, and the single oxygen percentage control lever could the necessary 'breath by breath' adjustment of the gas mixture be effected. Other important factors in successful use of the technique were that it was confined to robustly healthy patients, that they had the advantage of extra vital capacity from the sitting position, and that the airway was kept free. Any impedance of airway would add obstructive anoxia to iatrogenic as well as imposing stress on the circulation from respiratory efforts against resistance. A means commonly employed to overcome airway resistance, especially that due to partial nasal obstruction, was to increase gas delivery pressure and spring load the exhale valve to a corresponding level. This continuous positive pressure assisted inspiration, thereby increasing tidal volume and uptake of anaesthetic agents. Expiratory resistance was not significantly damaging if the procedure were brief, the anaesthetic light and the patient healthy. The Demand Flow apparatus was highly prized for this facility—but use of intermittent positive pressure is now recognized to be a sounder means of achieving the same end.

As techniques involving hypoxia and continuous positive pressure are no longer employed, it is not necessary to use the demand flow machine. Nasal administration can be effected with a modern continuous flow apparatus by attaching the nasal mask or inhaler to the Magill circuit in the manner to be described. The deficiencies of Demand Flow apparatus in relation to unreliability of the oxygen percentage scale have been well documented—(Parbrook 1964)—there is, however, a more cogent objection to its use, its unfamiliarity to the modern anaesthetist. Accustomed as he is to reading individual gas flows direct, and to having a reservoir bag by which he can estimate tidal ventilation and give respiratory assistance at need, the modern anaesthetist is hampered by the classical apparatus. The old machine virtually ties the anaesthetist to one method and prevents him from making use of the refinements of technique to which he is accustomed.

The sitting position

The other feature of 'nasal gas' which is objectionable is the sitting position of the patient. This arose from tradition and has been retained out of convenience but it is becoming increasingly evident that it should be abandoned and the horizontal posture used instead. Most of the points which might favour the retention of the sitting position have been set out by Coplans (Coplans 1962)—these are of greatest significance where the techniques of the modern anaesthetist are not used in dealing with airway problems. Difference in vital capacity and tidal respiration between the patient sitting and supine can be obviated by gentle assistance to breathing using intermittent positive pressure. Regurgitation of gastric contents is neither certainly prevented by sitting up nor necessarily caused by recumbency—it is, however, possible to manage this mishap more effectively in the recumbent patient than in the seated patient.

The important argument for the abandonment of the upright position relates to the risk of circulatory collapse or syncope causing death. The classical article of J. G. Bourne (Bourne 1957) described the risks plainly and unequivocally, it is a pity that his work seems to have been misunderstood. Bourne collected by questionnaire to dentists and anaesthetists, accounts of cases in which patients suffered complications chiefly suggestive of brain damage or of severe circulatory collapse, in association with administration of 'Dental Gas' in the chair. He postulated that these were due to fainting, occurring in a patient in the upright position, the unconsciousness resulting from cerebral anaemia being usually mistaken for the onset of general anaesthesia—and ignored. He described a clinical experiment on a patient receiving nitrous oxide in the sitting position. A precipitous drop in blood pressure which resulted passed unnoticed by the anaesthetist, but was detected by the use of a physiological monitor of blood pressure. This provided convincing evidence of the ease with which fainting can be overlooked by an expert anaesthetist who is watching for it, and can thereby result in serious deficiency of cerebral perfusion as a result of the upright position being maintained.

Whether it be due to fainting or to some other mechanism, the fact is that a severe fall of blood pressure occasionally occurs in the course of general anaesthesia. Even with the patient horizontal this may be serious, if the patient is in the sitting position or the supine reclining position the resultant lack of cerebral perfusion or failure of coronary circulation may be fatal or may lead to irreversible harm to the patient. Some small idea of the lethal potential of this condition is obtained when one measures the blood pressure after a patient who has fainted has been laid flat. It is not uncommon to find that the systolic pressure is as low as 50 mmHg even when recovery is under way. Bourne emphasized that the seriousness of the condition stems from its being potentially fatal, not from any frequency of occurrence. He emphasized that it is a rare event. The publication a few months later (Goldman *et al.* 1958), of an account of 100 consecutive cases in which blood pressure was maintained despite the sitting position, epitomizes a common attitude to this condition—the anaesthetist who has not experienced it tends to deny its occurrence, an attitude reminiscent of that formerly held by some anaesthetists towards primary circulatory arrest with chloroform.

Airway maintenance

Avoidance of airway obstruction is fundamental in any form of general anaesthesia and has always received emphasis in dental cases

Chapter 3

because the dentist's role in keeping a clear airway during extractions under open anaesthesia has been an important feature of dental school teaching. Many dentists have gained a high degree of skill in placement of mouth packs and in effecting support of the mandible to avoid obstruction to respiration and soiling of the air passages during extractions under nasally administered anaesthesia. The skills of the dentist have been instrumental in making the technique very safe, but the modern anaesthetist who participates in this field tends to be perturbed at delegating entirely to the surgeon a task so important as airway maintenance—and herein lies a further objection to the sitting position of the patient. With the patient upright in the chair, airway protection is of necessity carried out somewhat blindly—the insertion of a laryngoscope is not easy, therefore inspection of the pharynx and glottis will not be readily performed. The supine position, on the other hand, makes laryngoscopy and pharyngeal suction under vision much easier (Fig. 8). The anaesthetist feels more secure if he has ready access to the airway at need.

It is not intended at this stage to make comparison of endotracheal and 'open' techniques—that will be done when non-endotracheal methods have been fully described. The point is made now, by way of clarification, that the important place for nasal administration of

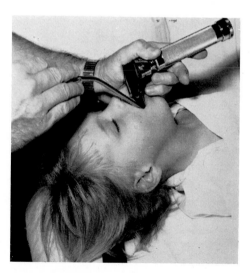

Fig. 8.   The anaesthetist should be prepared at any time to insert a laryngo-scope and perform pharyngeal suction under vision.

anaesthesia is in extractions in children, chiefly of deciduous teeth. Those with experience of dental anaesthesia know that difficulty with open techniques tends to arise in resistant adults. The specialist anaesthetist knows that adults can be dealt with by endotracheal intubation using modern methods, with minimal difficulty and with very little risk of significant complications. He is also keenly aware of course that endotracheal intubation in small children may be technically more difficult and that it carries risks of its own which cannot be lightly dismissed. In describing non-endotracheal methods therefore, emphasis will be placed on their use in children—especially small children having deciduous extractions, for it is here that the technique is fully justifiable as being the best available for the patient in almost any circumstances. A general description will first be given, and then each section of the procedure will be examined in detail. Most important, the various problems which commonly arise in use of this technique will be studied from the point of view of their recognition and management. In the course of this it is hoped that the justification of the method in the eyes of the specialist anaesthetist will emerge, as he recognizes that this type of procedure is not merely a hangover from former times but rather constitutes a soundly based method for handling brief anaesthetic administrations for surgery in the mouth, especially in small children.

NON-ENDOTRACHEAL TECHNIQUE

The anaesthetic apparatus which is employed for this is a standard continuous flow gas machine of the Boyle type, with the usual accessories (Fig. 9). The circuit is the Magill, with a reservoir bag at gas delivery from which a breathing tube leads to the face mask or nosepiece (Fig. 10). The patient lies supine upon a horizontal operating table: after intravenous induction with methohexitone, inhalation anaesthesia is effected using nitrous oxide and oxygen supplemented by halothane. The oxygen content of the mixture is never less than 20 per cent, usually 30 per cent or higher. Nasal breathing is established, the dentist places mouth packs according to the usual practice and proceeds to extraction of teeth. Volatile supplement is withdrawn early, and nitrous oxide turned off as the extractions are completed. Packs are placed over bleeding sockets, the patient turned into the lateral position, placed on a trolley and wheeled to a recovery area.

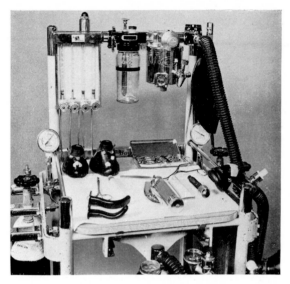

Fig. 9.   A continuous flow apparatus of the 'Boyle' type is in routine use
in the out-patient dental theatre.

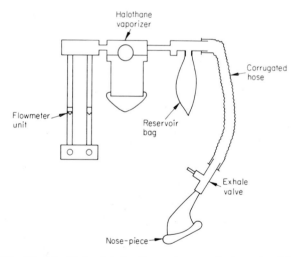

Fig. 10.   The Magill circuit is familiar to the anaesthetist and satisfactory
for nasal administration of nitrous oxide or for a short endotracheal
anaesthetic.

Agents and apparatus

The agents mentioned—methohexitone sodium for intravenous induction, and nitrous oxide and oxygen with halothane supplement—are named because they are customarily used: they are familiar to anaesthetists and appear to give satisfactory results. It should not be felt in any way that they are the correct or only agents. If an anaesthetist wishes for a particularly smooth induction in some case, thiopentone may be chosen. For a particularly quick recovery—propanidid may be the choice. The intention throughout is to describe techniques as illustrating matters of principle, many matters of detail are quite flexible.

The anaesthetic apparatus described is felt to be not entirely satisfactory on account of conflicting aims. The Goldman nose-piece was modified, for example, to achieve flexibility allowing easy change from nosepiece to full face mask or to endotracheal adapter (Figs. 11, 12 and 13). A disadvantage is that dead space is unduly great. A further important consideration is provision for venting of waste gases: two methods have been tried. The Enderby gas exhaust ventilation valve (Enderby 1972) placed in the Magill circuit (Fig. 14) retains the advantage of a rebreathing bag which is visible to the surgeon, as an indicator of airway patency and ventilation. This arrangement increases dead space however, and makes establishment and maintenance of inhalational anaesthesia more difficult in children.

An alternative is to use, with the Magill circuit, a Rubens valve on the nose-piece (Fig. 15). To the exhale limb of this, the exhaust hose is adapted by a plastic sleeve. Caution is needed in case compression of the bag causes the exhale valve to stay in the closed position.

Induction

Intravenous induction is strongly recommended but with one major proviso—the anaesthetist should be sufficiently skilful for this to be safe, which entails more than mere technical skill in performance of venepuncture. The anaesthetist who employs intravenous induction in children needs to be skilled in all aspects of airway maintenance and protection and in assistance and control of respiration. The younger the patients involved, the more important is this point. The modern anaesthetist is familiar with the use of intravenous induction and neuromuscular blockade, a practice which engenders a positive

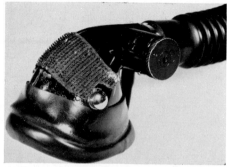

Fig. 11. The built-in exhale valve on the Goldman nose-piece diminishes dead space but makes change to a full face mask less easy.

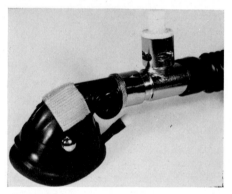

Fig. 12. This Goldman nose-piece has been modified by fitting a universal female taper and blanking off the exhale valve.

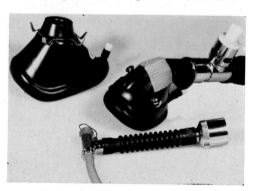

Fig. 13. The modified nose-piece is readily interchangeable, on a standard exhale valve mount, with a full face mask or an endotracheal adapter.

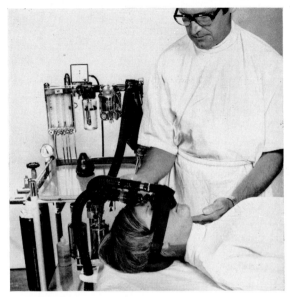

Fig. 14. The Enderby Gas Exhaust valve in use with the Magill circuit.

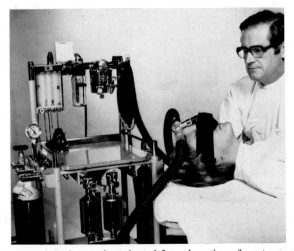

Fig. 15. A Rubens valve adapted for exhausting of waste gases.

approach to respiratory problems. Any respiratory depression following intravenous induction is immediately remedied by intermittent positive pressure breathing using a face mask.

There are practitioners however who are skilled at administration of 'nasal gas' to children, but who lack such training and experience in positive airway management. Such people should not be encouraged lightly to adopt the practice of intravenous induction in children. Problems with airway during recovery may be accentuated by use of intravenous instead of gaseous induction and this should receive consideration if a change to intravenous induction is proposed.

An intravenous induction which is smoothly performed is most impressive, but smoothness is achieved only by technical skill combined with sound teamwork—attention to detail is important. A vein on the dorsum of the hand is usually chosen, a venous tourniquet having been applied, and the hand and arm stabilized against the operating table top (Fig. 16). The use of a mechanical venous tourniquet (Fig. 17) has advantages over reliance upon manual pressure by an assistant: the latter is more likely to move the skin over the site of venepuncture as pressure is released, dislodging

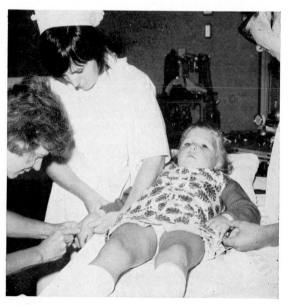

Fig. 16. Although this child appears to be unworried by the intravenous injection it is advisable to have a nurse holding the patient's free hand.

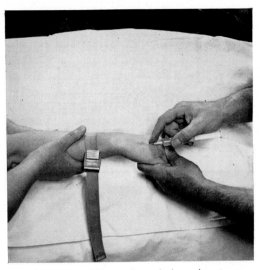

Fig. 17. When a venous tourniquet is used, the assistant can concentrate fully on holding the arm steady.

the needle, and there may also be a simultaneous partial loss of control of the arm in a child who is not co-operative. An assistant holding the arm must be taught the importance of firmly stabilizing the arm without hurting the patient, and of maintaining the position while the venous tourniquet is released—it is also essential that this assistant concentrate her full visual attention on the site of venepuncture—any movement of her eyes away will almost inevitably be accompanied by movement of her grip. The needle must be sharp if venepuncture is to be achieved readily. Disposable or 'single use' needles have made this more easily attainable. Important features in selecting a suitable needle are not only the sharpness of its point, but also the size of its lumen which should be sufficiently large to allow easy aspiration of blood.

The points of most disposable needles are easily deformed by mere contact with any hard surface, be it a metal dish, a glass ampule, or even the plastic needle sheath, and any 'turning' of the point tends to defeat the best efforts at venepuncture. In relation to technique of venepuncture, it is often recommended that the skin be punctured by a quick movement, but this practice is not conducive to precision. It is better to touch the needle point on the skin, gently reassure the patient, then penetrate the skin. The penetration is generally not more disturbing than the contact; if any movement is made this occurs on mere contact and no harm is done. When the point of the needle is correctly placed in the vein as verified by aspiration of blood, the needle hub is stabilized against the skin, usually by the thumb of the hand with which the anaesthetist is holding the patient's fingers (Fig. 18). The initial injection is made tentatively, watching the site of the needle point for swelling which would suggest extravenous injection: any doubt about placement of the needle may be resolved by injection of a test dose. If this is seen to act within fifteen seconds, the injection may be presumed to be intravenous and may safely be continued, an appropriate dose being injected more rapidly. To avoid the formation of a haematoma at the injection site it is important immediately to strap over it with adhesive tape a pad of dry gauze or cotton wool.

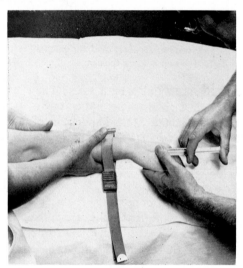

Fig. 18.   The arm must be stable while the injection is made.

Inhalation induction

Induction of general anaesthesia by breathing of nitrous oxide can be a fairly pleasant procedure, but the patient usually experiences at least some hallucinatory phenomena, auditory and sometimes visual, and these are occasionally remembered as being extremely unpleasant. It is difficult to avoid completely the occurrence of some sense of suffocation on application of the breathing mask. These are the main considerations which lead one to recommend and practise intravenous induction routinely, but in the occasional patient it will be for some reason either impossible or undesirable to effect it—thus the anaesthetist should have some skill in inhalational induction of anaesthesia. In describing this, which was the classical method of induction of dental anaesthesia, the relevance of certain features of dental anaesthetic teaching deserves consideration.

Nasal breathing

In dental anaesthetic teaching the nasal inhaler has usually been used from the outset, because of a need to 'establish nasal breathing' early. Controversy existed over the best means of achieving this—whether, for example, the mouth should be covered by an 'inert' cover such as a pack, or by a mouth cover which delivered gas mixture—there was however, general agreement that early establishment of nasal breathing was an important key to success. Experience in administration of nitrous oxide as a form of sedation or conscious analgesia has convinced one that in the conscious or semi-conscious patient there is some significance in establishment of nasal breathing—in teaching the patient to maintain an oropharyngeal closure when the mouth is open. Once consciousness is abolished, however, as by intravenous medication, there can be no relevance in these considerations at all. Once consciousness is lost, the placement of the mouth pack and the use of intermittent positive pressure through a nasal mask will be the determinants of nasal breathing. It is for this reason that in descriptions of induction or establishing of inhalational anaesthesia free use is made of the oropharyngeal airway and the full mask: the classical consideration is purposely ignored.

Hypoxic gas mixture

There have been various phases in this practice of which a brief resumé is therefore given. The first phase involved 'straight' nitrous oxide by single dose inhalation with a gross brief hypoxia and will not be further considered. There have been various schools of thought about anaesthesia using unsupplemented nitrous oxide and oxygen—an early one restricted the oxygen to about ten per cent for maintenance of anaesthesia. After the physiological significance of the shape of the dissociation curve of oxyhaemoglobin was recognized, the reasonable limit was put up to sixteen per cent oxygen for maintenance of anaesthesia, as below this level there would be rapid falling off in saturation of haemoglobin with oxygen. The rather naïve feature of these was the tacit assumption that a sufficiently high oxygen percentage according to certain physiological calculations was a safeguard against hypoxia. Having regard to the likelihood of some degree of airway restriction occurring during the anaesthetic administration, it is more logical to insist always upon a significant excess of oxygen above the minimum theoretically necessary for safety. A debt to one's predecessors is gratefully acknowledged. In the Melbourne Dental School, some thirty years ago and more, Geoffrey Kaye was campaigning against deliberate use of hypoxia and encouraging use of volatile supplementary agents, at first ether, and later trichlorethylene (Kaye *et al.* 1946). For quite some years the phenomena of cyanosis, jactitation, eccentric eyeballs and anoxic rigidity have existed, as regular events, only in the memory of senior dental staff and curiously, until a few years ago, in student lectures.

One consideration is still relevant: the advisability of using pure nitrous oxide at any stage of inhalational induction of anaesthesia in a child. There are those who suggest that it is safe to start with pure nitrous oxide provided the face mask is held 'off the face' and provided that a sufficient flow of oxygen is added to give not less than twenty per cent before the mask is applied to the face. Although this is efficacious its potential dangers deserve emphasis because of variations in conditions. Any mixture of nitrous oxide and air contains less than twenty per cent oxygen: if the nitrous oxide has an effect, the patient must have been subjected to oxygen restriction. When a continuous flow machine is used the nitrous oxide may flow at about ten litres per minute; the intermittent flow apparatus set to deliver at three to five mmHg pressure may deliver thirty or forty litres per minute. Using it in this way it is not uncommon to see some cyanosis of the lips in a child before the mask is put on the face.

Against these arguments, the experienced anaesthetist points out that smoothness of induction, in terms of freedom from breath holding and spasm, is an advantage of using pure nitrous oxide which outweighs its theoretical dangers. This is a decision which is in the hands of the anaesthetist, but he should have the clearest possible idea of precisely what his patient is breathing at all times.

Technique of gas induction

The outstanding subjective feature of inhaling nitrous oxide is auditory hyperacusis—there should be general silence during induction. The anaesthetist should speak quietly to the child, reassuring him specifically about noises, and about the sensation of falling which may be experienced. The mask should be held off the face until consciousness is obtunded slightly, whatever gas mixture is given. It is desirable to avoid giving halothane while a child is still actively resisting, but this may be sometimes necessary. Should an inhalational mixture be used to subdue a struggling child, the oxygen content of the mixture should never be below about thirty per cent, to allow for the increased metabolic rate, and flow rate should be sufficiently great to minimize rebreathing which might otherwise lead to increased levels of carbon dioxide—a source of danger in halothane anaesthesia. A significant advantage of using inhalational anaesthesia from the start is the absence of respiratory depression effect from the intravenous agent. There is strongly suggestive evidence that the hallucinatory and other psychological phenomena of induction by nitrous oxide are so unpleasant to some patients as to produce a degree of nervous or mental upset later (Bergström *et al* 1968). Although one is not aware of evidence that this occurs in children it deserves mention as a further point supporting the increased use of intravenous induction.

ESTABLISHMENT OF INHALATIONAL ANAESTHESIA

Following intravenous induction, the anaesthetist moves to the head of the table, at the patient's left side and places a mask over the nose, or nose and mouth, with a flow of the order of oxygen two litres per minute and nitrous oxide six litres per minute. The exhale valve is closed at this stage so that a hand on the reservoir bag of the anaesthetic apparatus may be used to provide gentle intermittent inflation of the lungs (Fig. 19). This tests the patency of the airways and the fit of the mask, and assists in overcoming hesitant breathing and minor spasm. Respiratory assistance at this stage should be minimal and is directed merely towards encouraging onset of rhythmic breathing by the patient. Until the exhale valve is opened, expiration is allowed by

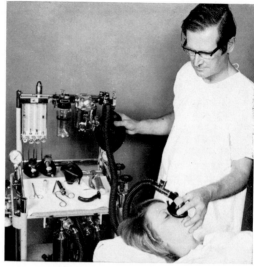

Fig. 19.   The anaesthetist's hand on the rebreathing bag can test the patency of the airway and provide gentle assistance to breathing.

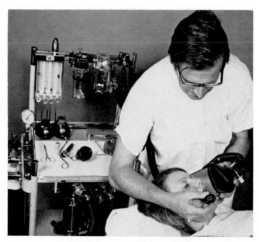

Fig. 20.   Any restriction of nasal airway is an indication for insertion of a Guedel oropharyngeal airway.

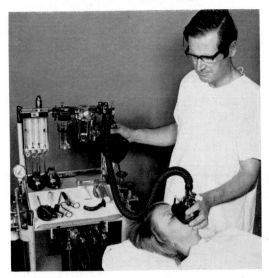

Fig. 21. The full face mask can readily replace the nose-piece at need.

raising a corner of the mask by tilting it. Testing and maintaining the patency of air passages at every point is absolutely vital. At this stage free nasal breathing is sought—if it is not absolutely free, an oro-pharyngeal airway of the Guedel pattern is inserted early, and a full face mask replaces the nasal mask if necessary (Figs. 20 and 21).

Halothane is introduced as soon as respiration through a free airway is established, except that the insertion of an oro-pharyngeal airway to relieve partial obstruction to breathing may be better delayed until the patient has tolerated at least a few breaths of halothane vapour. The concentration is increased, usually to three per cent, or even four per cent, fairly rapidly, but it is held at that level only until anaesthesia is of adequate depth, as suggested by quiescence of the patient, regular respiration and by lack of response to firm finger tip pressure on the angle of the mandible. The concentration of halothane is then reduced, and the change to nasal administration is carried out.

The nose-piece is placed over the nose only, the oral airway is removed and the mandible supported firmly (Fig. 22). A check is made of the adequacy of respiration and airway by observation of the excursion of the reservoir bag and of chest and tracheal movement of the patient. A poor airway at this stage, as manifest by chest retraction, tracheal tug, and poor bag excursion demands immediate action to relieve it. The cushion of the nasal mask may be placed too high and occlude the nares, or increased extension of the head and forward lift to the mandible may be necessary. If airway obstruction is not relieved by attention to such simple points, it is desirable to perform direct laryngoscopy (Fig. 8, p. 32) to ascertain the cause of the problem. The act of insertion of the curved McIntosh laryngoscope generally gives immediate relief of the obstruction by lifting forward the tongue, and further management of the problem is discussed in detail shortly. Once nasal breathing is established in a satisfactory manner, the next step is that the dentist opens the mouth, inserts a mouth prop or gag and places a mouth pack (Fig. 23). The integrity of the airway should be immediately checked again before any extraction of teeth is undertaken. If this is not done, then the position is likely to emerge that one is trying to deal with an obstructed airway with the mouth full of blood. It is most important that airway obstruction following initial opening of the mouth and placement of a mouth pack is not overlooked. The immediate treatment is to adjust the mouth pack by pulling it forward, if this is not successful, a laryngoscope should be introduced—this frees the airway and exposes the whole situation. Certain decisions need to be made on the basis of what is found, a consideration of what surgery is to be done, the capabilities of the surgeon and the age and general state of the patient.

If the operation planned is extractions in one quadrant of the mouth in a very young child and the airway obstruction is partial, the correct decision may well be to ventilate the patient using an oral airway, then to replace the pack and prop and proceed with the extractions speedily, even in the presence of partial airway obstruction. In the case of an older child to have extractions in all four quadrants of the mouth and especially if the dentist is not very experienced, the correct procedure may be to administer a muscle relaxant and proceed with endotracheal intubation. One's attitude is of importance here—endotracheal intubation and the non-endotracheal technique are merely alternative ways of giving an anaesthetic—the more suitable one is selected. It is important to avoid the concept that airway obstruction arising during an 'open' type anaesthetic represents a failure or mishap, and intubation an 'emergency measure' to overcome the problem.

The chief means of maintaining a clear pharyngeal airway is extension of the head and holding of the jaw forward which should be

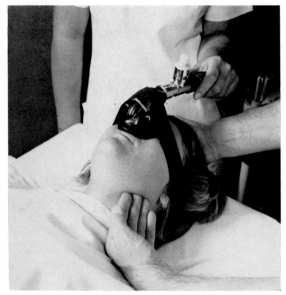

Fig. 22.   Shows a means of effecting support on the mandible with a
minimum of effort.

performed by the anaesthetist. It is most easily carried out by placing
the back of one hand on the corresponding shoulder of the patient,
fingers straight at the inter-phalangeal joints but flexed at the meta-
carpophalangeal joints, finger tips supporting the angle of the jaw
(Fig. 22). The other hand is placed on top of the head to maintain the
extended position. Airway maintenance in this way necessitates delegating the task of holding the nosepiece to a nurse—if the head
harness is not adequate. There will still be cases in which an adequate
airway will not be maintained by these simple measures—laryngoscopy will generally reveal an obvious cause such as excessive lymphoid tissue or occasionally a deformed epiglottis which makes
abnormal contact with the posterior pharyngeal wall and blocks the
breathing. Trial of various head positions under vision may reveal
one which frees the airway, otherwise a nasopharyngeal or nasotracheal airway may be found necessary. Other rare causes such as
laryngeal polyp may be found—such cases will be dealt with by the
anaesthetist secundum artem.

MOUTH PACKING

Careful mouth packing is essential to the success of the procedure and certain principles need to be observed in carrying it out, but the view that meticulous mouth packing is the solution to all airway problems in anaesthesia or sedation by non-endotracheal methods has sometimes been rather exaggerated. The concept of a mouth pack placed over the dorsum of the tongue and forming a curtain or partition between mouth and pharynx is not tenable, it is too difficult to place such a pack successfully, without obstructing breathing. The method used is based broadly on what has been well described by various authors, but particularly by Coplans and Barton (1964). The principles are:

1. For safety's sake, the individual pack should be too large to be placed entirely in the mouth: any pack small enough to disappear in the mouth may sooner or later impact in the larynx, with awkward if not fatal results.

2. Before working on one side of the mouth the prop is placed on the other, the tongue pulled forwards and laterally against the prop, and a pack inserted with its back end behind the molar teeth, its front end preventing mouth breathing, its middle reaching from roof to floor of the mouth (Fig. 23).

3. This pack will be changed if its becoming blood soaked or soiled necessitates it, the sucker is used during the change, and the laryngoscope too, if indicated.

4. When changing to the opposite side of the mouth, the mouth pack is removed, wiping the operative area clear on the way, and a fresh pack is placed over bleeding sockets, with one of its ends protruding. The mouth prop is changed to this side, then another pack placed with its end behind the molar teeth as described for the first side (Figs. 24 and 25).

5. At the conclusion, a pack is inserted on each side over bleeding sockets, and an oro-pharyngeal airway between them if needed (Fig. 26).

Various materials may be used for packs, 'combine dressing' or Gamgee, in which the gauze should adequately cover the wool, and individual packs should be long, plastic sponge packs, which should

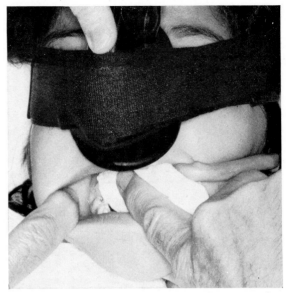

Fig. 23. In preparation for surgery, a mouth gag has been inserted and a pack placed, so as to protect the pharynx while extractions are performed on the right side of the mouth.

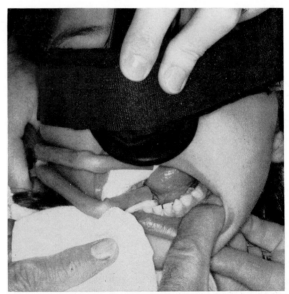

Fig. 24. For surgery on the second side, the mouth gag is inserted with a pack placed to protect the sockets. The mouth has been opened and the dentist is ready to place a mouth pack on the left side.

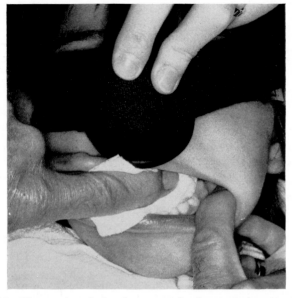

Fig. 25.   The mouth pack placed to protect the pharynx during extractions
on the left side of the mouth.

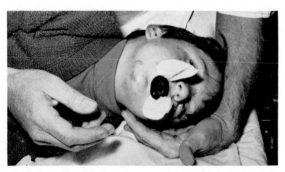

Fig. 26.   When extractions have involved both sides of the mouth, it may
be convenient to insert an airway between packs.

be autoclaved between uses, or gauze packs which should be of good
quality soft gauze. One purposely avoids favouring a particular
material or a precise method, to emphasize that packing is not 'the
be all and end all' of airway protection, that what is more important

is observation and care by an anaesthetist who is prepared to take appropriate early action as described to forestall serious complications.

INTRAVENOUS ANAESTHESIA

This deserves mention, if only because it is widely practised: it is not recommended. The idea of using an intravenous anaesthetic such as thiopentone, or more recently methohexitone, as a sole agent to maintain general anaesthesia for surgery is not new. It was common practice in the mid 1940s for many types of surgical procedure, but has largely fallen into disrepute. This is because of recognition of the fact that maintenance of a state of general anaesthesia by most intravenous agents for more than a short period leads to problems of high dosage, with undue respiratory and circulatory depression, as well as providing as a rule, mediocre conditions for the surgeon. Intravenous anaesthesia will be further discussed in Part III under intravenous sedation, as it is often difficult to distinguish these two methods.

The principal reasons for its popularity are patient acceptance of the technique, which is excellent, and simplicity of the method from the view point of the anaesthetist. Barbiturates give a very pleasant induction, and if the procedure is brief and dosage not too great, recovery is associated with a marked euphoria. The actual administration of the anaesthetic requires only a syringe and needle. Safe administration however needs an anaesthetist present with all the apparatus required for aspiration of the pharynx under vision, administration of oxygen by intermittent positive pressure and endotracheal intubation. Disadvantages are the inevitable respiratory depression—if the anaesthesia is at all adequate—difficulty of airway maintenance and liability to laryngospasm. These, coupled with very poor operating conditions in which the patient is liable to move, phonate or even cry out as extractions are performed, lead one to condemn this except as a method of convenience for limited use by very skilled personnel. If introduced as a teaching technique it could well repeat many mistakes of 'nasal gas'—putting a premium on speed of operation.

OPEN ANAESTHESIA

The general problem

The importance has been stressed in this description, of looking for and dealing with airway problems. The specialist anaesthetist trained in modern concepts wishes to be at all times in control of the situation relative to his patient. A few common problems will therefore be examined in an endeavour to show that this technique, properly carried out, allows the anaesthetist to be in full control. Some points should be made however before embarking on detail, concerning the basic safety of out-patient management of dental cases with general anaesthesia. It is sometimes difficult for the specialist anaesthetist who is not usually involved with dental cases to accept the fact that non-endotracheal anaesthesia on an out-patient basis for extraction of teeth can be a safe procedure. This attitude stems chiefly from an ignorance of the precise nature of the surgery. The important features of dental extractions and restorative work, with very few exceptions, are flexibility in actual performance and a high degree of freedom from serious post-operative morbidity. These are the major considerations which lead one to use a simple anaesthetic technique for most deciduous extractions, and to perform many dental procedures on an out-patient basis. If consideration is made only of straightforward exodontia and restorative dental work, a feature of dental surgery is that it is not essential to the patient's safety that once started, the surgery should be completed forthwith. This fact, that extraction or restoration of teeth can be immediately abandoned or interrupted without serious harm is a major safety factor in out-patient management of general anaesthesia for dentistry. There can never be any justification for continuing with a dental general anaesthetic in unsatisfactory conditions—the surgery can, and sometimes must, be interrupted or even abandoned at short notice.

The other important factor relating to the surgery is the incidence and likely nature of post-operative surgical complications such as haemorrhage. Haemorrhage following extraction of teeth is difficult to overlook, it can be recognized by a lay person looking in the mouth, the 'first aid' treatment—biting on a wad of clean linen—is simple to teach and apply, and this is usually the definitive treatment.

This perhaps gives some insight into the reasons why specialist anaesthetists whose activities are largely confined to dealing with cases of major surgery, have a very different viewpoint from that of anaesthetists who regularly deal with dental cases, who find them mainly straightforward and trouble-free employing the simplest of methods. The major problem which arises in maintenance of open general anaesthesia for extractions is airway obstruction—and the closely related problem of soiling of the pharynx and air passages with blood and other foreign material. Learning to deal with these problems is a practical exercise, but some important features deserve mention.

The non-endotracheal technique has its greatest safety when extractions are performed in one quadrant only, there is no changing sides involved. The mouth pack which protects the pharynx may be placed, as described earlier, beside the tongue, with its end behind the molar teeth. In this place it is least likely to cause obstruction and can give effective protection to the airway against soiling. On completion of extraction, it is either used to wipe out the operative field and replaced with a clean pack, or it may be merely placed over the sockets, an airway may be inserted beside it if needed.

The airway problem

When extractions are to be performed on two sides of the mouth, a common problem is that airway control is threatened by some surgical difficulty—it may be brisk haemorrhage or it may be that a tooth is broken off and extra time is needed to look for the roots—it may be some combination of these. If the nasal airway is quite free, then maintenance of anaesthesia may present no problem. However when nasal breathing is restricted, there may be problems with the patient from two factors: firstly, a threat of hypoxia and secondly, lightening of anaesthesia. Simple definitive action is needed to overcome this. Dry packs are placed over all bleeding sockets, an oro-pharyngeal airway is inserted, and the patient ventilated and anaesthesia deepened through the airway thus provided. As auxiliary measures to effect this it may be necessary to insert a laryngoscope to clear the pharynx and glottis of foreign material under vision: it may be desirable to turn the patient into the lateral position, and perhaps slightly head down. After some two minutes there should be a dramatic diminution of bleeding—partly from mere pressure of packs, but also because with adequate airway and anaesthesia, there will be no venous congestion from straining against airway obstruction, and no coughing or laryngospasm. The emphasis here is on prevention of aspiration—the anaesthetist must also, of course, be able to deal with threatened or actual aspiration of foreign material be it blood, vomitus or any other: this is described fully in a later chapter (Chapter 5, p. 63) in connection with complications of general anaesthesia.

With sufficient description having been given to convey some idea of the value of non-endotracheal methods of general anaesthesia for dentistry, some comparisons will now be undertaken in an effort to establish what is its place in the out-patient general anaesthesia clinic. Following this examination of techniques, consideration will be given to management of the out-patient clinic in regard to selection and briefing of patients, and management of recovery.

CHAPTER 4
CHOICE OF TECHNIQUE

In the two preceding chapters an account has been given of endotracheal and of non-endotracheal techniques of general anaesthesia as they are applied in dentistry. In this chapter a comparison will be made of the efficacy and safety of these two methods, but certain points must first be made clear. It is not a question of deciding that one method is 'right' and the other 'wrong', but rather of recognizing that each has its place, and trying to determine what is the utility of each method. Further, it is important to recognize that many factors must be considered in making a sound decision about the best technique in any given situation, that these include not only the patient and the operation, but also the environment and various aspects of the skill of anaesthetist and dentist. Considerations in this last category are sometimes regarded askance by the specialist anaesthetist as being compromises which are necessitated merely by a situation which is far from ideal—this attitude is not justifiable, and as it involves important matters of principle it will be considered in all its implications. The glib statement that, because the operation is in the mouth, and therefore interferes with the airway, endotracheal anaesthesia should always be used in dentistry overlooks important points.

LIMITATIONS OF ENDOTRACHEAL TECHNIQUE

Such protection as an endotracheal tube provides is effective only during the time that it is correctly placed. There is a period before intubation when the air passages are unprotected in the unconscious patient, as well as a recovery period following removal of the tube, during both of these, the tube gives no protection to the patient against risks of aspiration of foreign material or obstruction of breathing.

In the case of dental procedures, a more profound level of anaesthesia or of neuromuscular blockade may be needed for intubation than is needed for the surgery. Prior to the insertion of an endotracheal tube the patient's safety is dependent upon the anaesthetist's ability to take definitive steps to relieve any threat of aspiration or obstruction. Following extubation, safety of the airway basically depends upon resumption of activity of protective reflexes, aided by a suitable posture and upon supervision—for a limited time by the anaesthetist—the duty being then delegated to the recovery room nurse. The anaesthetist who has the safety of his patient at heart will try to ensure that the recovery period is as brief and as safe as possible. If the operation is essentially brief and requires only light general anaesthesia, the anaesthetist may do his patient a disservice by intubation when he can, as already emphasized, remain in control of the patient's airway during the surgery, supervising its protection and being prepared to intervene effectively at need. When the operation is such that this intervention is not prevented, then a non-endotracheal method can be much safer, because the recovery period will generally be quicker and more straightforward if a tube has not been inserted. When one further considers the complications inherent in endotracheal intubation when used on small children, the case for open anaesthetic methods for deciduous extractions is very strong. In adults the method deserves consideration when extractions are straightforward and are being performed on an out-patient by an expert dentist.

It is difficult to argue this point with the well trained young anaesthetic specialist—to whom endotracheal is right and all else wrong. One needs to introduce him to an enlightened out-patient dental theatre and let him see and practise the open methods. Here he may see and appreciate as if for the first time the remarkable efficacy of protective reflexes in the unpremedicated child who has a brief, light anaesthetic. He is encouraged to use the laryngoscope freely and frequently to expose the glottis and see for himself that there has been no soiling of the air passages. In the course of a few sessions he gains an appreciation of the airway problems of the lightly anaesthetized or recovering patient, and a mature assurance in their management.

Surgical opinions

The young anaesthetist, however, is not the only one who may need to be convinced about the virtues of various methods. The dentist who is skilled at exodontia, and has become very accustomed to expert general anaesthesia given by one particular method may have difficulty in appreciating the virtues of any other technique. One should be chary of giving an endotracheal anaesthetic for a protagonist of the open technique. He is likely to be a very quick exodontist, and may take some delight in completing his task so quickly that the anaesthetist is 'left squeezing the bag'. He will not hesitate to be critical of any nasal haemorrhage caused by the tube, nor to draw attention to the symptoms of sore throat or muscle pains after the event. There is another side to this—the oral surgeon who is a convert to insistence upon endotracheal anaesthesia on an in-patient basis being the correct, and therefore the 'only' form of general anaesthesia may also hold strong views. Having learned the virtues of full, free, unhurried access for surgical removal of teeth, he may be unwilling to countenance any departure from this. He knows and accepts the complications—or at least the discomforts associated with intubation, and expects his patient to put up with them. It is a pity if his enthusiasm leads to his demanding a tube for a very brief simple extraction of an anterior tooth, for example. The anaesthetist who gives dental anaesthetics should take the trouble to become skilled in both techniques and should be prepared to keep a very open mind, in this way he will usually be able to do what is best for the surgeon and even more important—the patient.

The non-specialist anaesthetist

In relation to dental anaesthesia, the attitude taken by the specialist anaesthetist tends to be that the only reason why open methods are still used is because the anaesthetist is incapable of passing a tube. It is hoped that what has already been said about techniques makes it clear that there are abundant justifications for use of non-endotracheal methods in many circumstances: but the question of anaesthetic administration by non-specialists still deserves consideration. Firstly, whatever may be ideal it will be some years at least before anaesthetists are trained in sufficient numbers to take over all anaesthetic administrations. Secondly, it is questionable if the services of the specialist are most urgently needed in the dental field: better perhaps to provide this with a sound practice to follow and let non-specialists do the work. This is a field par excellence where the cautious anaesthetist can safely opt out of the difficult case, whether before or during the surgery.

The statement about practitioners who are unable to intubate deserves comment. Of medical men who give dental anaesthetics, there will be fewer every year who are 'unable' to intubate because—for many years now—learning to pass an endotracheal tube has been a part of the training of most resident Medical Officers in hospitals. It is more accurate to say of many such practitioners that they are not very skilled in intubation. This being the case, they are obviously wise to avoid it if there is a suitable alternative. They are particularly wise to avoid intubation of children, and if working with a skilled exodontist, should rarely need to do this.

Whether in the field of anaesthesia, surgery or psychiatry, the specialist needs to do better than merely suggest an embargo on practice of these special branches by the non-specialist. A sounder scheme is—firstly to give a broad undergraduate education in the specialty, so that its potential is known. Undergraduate teaching which is carried on in the same environment as is specialist post-graduate teaching, makes education of the undergraduate more sound. The specialist should make a careful study of the areas in which the general practitioner is liable to be involved, with a view to delineation of sound practice.

AIRWAY CARE

In the field of out-patient dental anaesthesia, the specialist most needs to give precise guidance in regard to airway maintenance and protection, and the avoidance of aspiration of foreign material. These points have for many years received emphasis in dental school teaching relative to general anaesthesia, but anaesthetic practice has changed. In former times emphasis was on keeping out of trouble, on giving every possible aid to the patient's own reflexes and to spontaneous breathing. The modern anaesthetist is schooled in positive or aggressive airway maintenance and protection. The ultimate here is insertion of an endotracheal tube, but even where this is not used, or after it is removed, the modern anaesthetist tends to early positive action in relation to airway obstruction. He is very ready to apply a face mask and use gentle intermittent positive pressure ventilation to overcome, or even avert laryngospasm: his readiness to do this will, of course, be increased if his patient is in the supine or the lateral position, and easily accessible for laryngoscopy.

Early positive action to avert or minimize respiratory obstruction is a potent factor in avoidance of aspiration of foreign material into the air passages. If obstruction is allowed to persist, the resulting hypoxaemia builds up a strong respiratory drive: moving of a mouth pack may allow vigorous inspiration through the mouth past bleeding sockets, with a high risk of aspiration of débris, blood or even a pack (Constable 1964). Obstruction simultaneously aggravates haemorrhage by causing venous congestion, elevation of blood pressure and capillary dilatation, increasing the potential for aspiration. The associated lightening of the plane of anaesthesia makes vomiting likely—with a grave risk of inhalation of acid secretion or even food. Action has always been recommended and taken to reduce these dangers. The rule of fasting before general anaesthesia minimizes vomiting and its seriousness. Avoidance of general anaesthesia in patients with acute respiratory infections has been the rule because of liability to nasal obstruction, and to obstruction to breathing from laryngospasm and presence of secretions. Smooth anaesthesia with avoidance of spasm and vomiting makes for safety, likewise expert surgery in which haemorrhage is minimized and various sources of airway obstruction are avoided. If to these measures are added the supine position of the patient, and full use of the means of active airway maintenance and protection of the modern anaesthetist, then safety will be very great. Of perhaps greater importance is the fact that teaching is facilitated. Teaching the risks of airway obstruction and the readiness with which this occurs in the unconscious patient is a task which is difficult, but is of great importance. As dental practitioners make increasing use of sedation techniques, it is vital that they learn in depth about airway obstruction and its management.

When laryngoscopy is readily used, the cause of any obstructive episode will never be in doubt and its management may be plainly demonstrated. If the dentist learns to use intermittent positive pressure breathing, he will be armed with the means to deal with laryngospasm and depression of breathing and will never hesitate to acknowledge the occurrence or even the threat of these, but will be able to proceed immediately to deal with them.

Anaesthetic management, and teaching and practice of airway maintenance, has always been extremely well performed in the good dental out-patient general anaesthetic clinic. If to this traditional excellence is added the equipment and methods of the modern anaesthetist, then dental anaesthesia can once again be in the forefront of teaching of basic methods of general anaesthesia.

CHAPTER 5
COMPLICATIONS OF ANAESTHESIA

The patient who undergoes general anaesthesia for dentistry is liable to any of the complications which may be associated with an anaesthetic, yet serious complications in practice are not common. Rather than attempting to deal exhaustively with complications it is intended to consider some of those which are liable to occur in dental practice and especially those of which the management is particularly important.

An increased use of endotracheal anaesthesia raises specific problems and some of these will be examined. The fact that non-endotracheal methods are commended makes it obligatory to consider the dangers of aspiration of foreign material into the air passages. This is dealt with in association with vomiting as a complication; post-anaesthetic vomiting is mentioned because of the importance of keeping this in a correct perspective. When circulatory arrest occurs in dental practice, the plan of action usually recommended for an operating theatre needs certain modifications which are outlined. Lastly certain rare complications are noted, to highlight the diffculty of keeping a reasonable sense of balance in teaching dental undergraduates about these.

COMPLICATIONS OF ENDOTRACHEAL INTUBATION

It is necessary to distinguish clearly between complications which are little more than a nuisance, and those which are potentially serious. Various structures may suffer trauma during endotracheal intubation and whereas trauma to the lips or tongue, or epistaxis from the anterior naris is rarely serious, any damage to the pharynx or larynx is of greater significance.

Laryngeal trauma may largely be avoided by careful, deliberate technique, and exercise of sound judgment in relation to the depth of anaesthesia or muscular relaxation necessary for intubation. The major difference between adults and children in relation to the significance of laryngeal trauma has aleady been mentioned (Chapter 2, page 26). Where an adult may suffer short lived hoarseness and sore throat, minor trauma in a child may be followed by severe stridor and threat of respiratory obstruction from sub-glottic oedema. Children under six years of age who have endotracheal anaesthesia need to be observed for not less than two hours post-operatively. Any sign of hoarseness or 'croup' is an indication for further observation, and for seeking signs of respiratory restriction, such as chest retraction or stridor on inspiration. If these are noted then treatment as for laryngo-tracheo-bronchitis should be instituted urgently.

Pharyngeal trauma varies in its degree of seriousness. In the course of intubation or throat packing it is not rare for the pharyngeal wall to be damaged by Magill forceps, or even for the pillar of the fauces to be penetrated. This latter event usually results from placing the laryngoscope incorrectly so that the pillar is stretched and vulnerable. Apart from short lived but embarrassing haemorrhage such tears are rarely followed by serious results, though post-operative follow up should be undertaken. An accident of more significance is that in which a tube inserted nasally appears in the pharynx in the submucous position having penetrated the mucous membrane of the posterior region of the lateral wall of the nasal cavity. If the recommendation is followed that the laryngoscope be inserted before introduction of the nasal tube the mishap will be recognized early. Treatment is directed to avoiding possible serious consequences of this misplacement of the tube, namely haemorrhage from the nasopharynx or surgical emphysema in the neck. Either of these may cause trouble if the tube is removed and the lungs inflated by application of a face mask, the correct treatment therefore is to leave the nasal tube where it is and pass an orotracheal tube forthwith. Should the patient need re-oxygenation first a face mask should be applied so that it kinks and blocks the tube projecting from the nose. Once an orotracheal airway is securely established, removal of the nasal tube and assessment of the damage can be deliberately carried out. This accident is rare, but the principles of the treatment should be noted. There are various circumstances in which attempts at nasal intubation should be abandoned and an orotracheal tube immediately inserted.

Whenever nasal intubation is undertaken, there should be available readily, an 'oral length' tube of appropriate size.

A prime reason for endotracheal intubation is to assure an un-obstructed airway—this is not invariably easy. Bronchospasm is a complication of anaesthesia which is a little more likely to occur, and very much more likely to be suspected, in cases in which the trachea is intubated under out-patient conditions when the patient is unpre-medicated and the anaesthesia light. When troublesome broncho-spasm occurs, one can often look back and find that the patient gives a history of bronchitis or asthma. It is difficult to decide however which of the numerous patients who admit to these conditions are likely to give trouble from this cause. Serious trouble is more likely in those patients who have some obvious signs or symptoms suggest-ing actual pulmonary impairment or damage. Examples are diminu-tion of chest movement and air entry, retraction of the mid to lower ribs on deep inspiration, copious sputum, persistent dyspnoea on moderate exertion as distinct from the varying disability imposed by intermittent bronchospasm. All these features should be sought in the preliminary history and examination of patients who are referred for consultation on account of a history of asthma. If such features are found, general anaesthesia should be avoided unless the nature of the surgery or of the patient overwhelmingly indicates its value.

The diagnosis of rapidly developing bronchospasm in the course of a general anaesthetic is not always easy, two errors are liable to occur. One is over-ready diagnosis on the occurrence of difficulty in infla-tion of the intubated patient. One should first ensure that the problem is not merely unduly light anaesthesia, while looking for technical faults related to the endotracheal tube. Kinking of the tube, hernia-tion of the inflated cuff and compression within the nasal passage are likely problems. It is useless to administer broncho-dilators for a blocked endotracheal tube, but the opposite error may lead to delay in treatment. Generally speaking, when obstruction arises shortly after placement of an endotracheal tube the tube should be removed immediately and an attempt made at inflation of the lungs by face mask. Exception to this rule will be made if there has been free haemorrhage in the nose or mouth, or if there has been considerable difficulty in placement of the tube. In these conditions it is reasonable to temporize while seeking to establish whether the tube is patent or obstructed.

The usual drug to use when diagnosis is established is aminophylline or isoprenaline given intravenously. Adrenaline is best avoided as it may have adverse cardiovascular effects, especially if hypoxia has been at all severe.

VOMITING

Vomiting occurring during anaesthesia is always a cause for alarm because of the risk of aspiration of vomited material into the air passages causing asphyxia. The dangers associated with this need to be precisely understood so that its potential seriousness is recognized, but its dangers are not exaggerated—particularly to the extent that an anaesthetist is persuaded to embark unnecessarily on complicated measures to deal with non-existent aspiration of material into the air passages.

Certain circumstances have an effect in determining what are the risks of aspiration of vomitus or other material in the course of a general anaesthetic.

1. **Fasting of the patient:**
   The presence of food, especially solids or milk in the stomach makes vomiting more dangerous than if there is fasting contents only. Not only is the likelihood of vomiting increased, but there is the added danger of impaction of solid matter in the air passages.

2. **Depth and duration of anaesthesia:**
   Vomiting or regurgitation under deep anaesthesia, or that associated with profound neuromuscular blockade, is potentially more serious because of lack of reflex protection against aspiration.

3. **Hypoxia:**
   Where a patient has become hypoxic as a result of a failure to recognize or to deal effectively with respiratory obstruction, the very strong respiratory drive which results may give rise to serious aspiration of vomitus or other material into the bronchial tree.

4. **State of health of the patient:**
   A patient suffering from disease or disability may be more at risk from aspiration of vomitus than is a healthy person.

These observations should make it evident that it is desirable that patients who are booked for general anaesthesia should be instructed to fast, and that efforts should be made, on the day of the procedure, to determine whether this has been observed. A rather extreme view is advanced in some text books on dental anaesthesia however, which so stress the rule of fasting as to imply that, if there is no food in the stomach, there is no risk from vomiting. The risk of vomiting is ever present, food in the stomach is merely one factor which increases its likelihood and the risks of aspiration. It has long been recognized that the risks of aspiration into the bronchial tree of material, whether vomitus, or operative débris, or secretions from the mouth, is increased by hypoxic episodes during general anaesthesia (Brock 1947)—hence the emphasis placed upon maintenance of a free airway at all stages of non-endotracheal administration of general anaesthesia for extractions (Chapter 3), and stress on the importance of the anaesthetist's being ready to perform laryngoscopy and pharyngeal toilet at the slightest suggestion of soiling of the pharynx.

Control of the depth of anaesthesia is important—anaesthesia for dental extractions does not require to be deep—the wise anaesthetist keeps patients light during open anaesthesia.

Complete reliance should not be placed on these points as a means of avoiding aspiration, but a consideration of them can assist in making a decision about management of the case where aspiration of vomit, blood or other foreign material is suspected. If vomiting under anaesthesia, or soiling of the pharynx occurs, action should be taken at the first suspicion of trouble. The patient should be turned immediately on to one side, the mouth sucked out and, unless anaesthesia is extremely light, laryngoscopy performed. If anaesthesia has been brief and smooth, and contamination of the pharynx is slight, the likelihood of aspiration is remote, and no further action is indicated, provided recovery proceeds normally. If the patient has had an episode of respiratory obstruction or if there is much foreign matter or vomit in the pharynx, the glottis should be observed after sucking out of the pharynx. A strong cough which produces only mucus is reassuring.

Only if the anaesthesia has been rather long or eventful, or if there is considerable contamination of the pharynx, would serious consideration be given to immediate intubation and tracheobronchial toilet. One would hesitate even over this, if it meant re-anaesthetizing a waking patient. If there is no frank airway obstruction, better to let the patient wake up, observing him closely, listening to breath sounds, also seeking any sign such as restlessness, slight cyanosis, or rapid pulse, which might be suggestive of bronchial obstruction, and to transfer the patient urgently to a general hospital if such signs are observed.

In the event of vomiting of solid food being followed by obvious airway obstruction, laryngoscopy should be performed. If this shows that solid or particulate material has been aspirated, then broncho-scopy may be necessary. This is a difficult situation if the anaesthetist cannot call on expert help: if forced into it he should take the bronchoscope and place it in the larynx before the laryngoscope is removed, and only then look through it. Aspiration of the trachea should be thoroughly carried out, and each main bronchus entered in turn and aspirated if contamination is seen. Oxygenation through the bronchoscope in the trachea should then be effected, if the patient's colour is satisfactory the instrument may be removed. The patient can be transferred to a general hospital for further management—only a minimum should be done in the emergency situation.

Post-operative vomiting

Vomiting as a post-operative complication is relatively common, but rarely serious. Management of the condition and especially the briefing of out-patients post-operatively must be such that the con-dition does not assume major significance unnecessarily, but should ensure that the occasional severe vomiting will be correctly handled. Parents of child patients should be warned almost to expect that the first drink taken may be vomited, and that the vomit may contain blood which has been swallowed. Their instructions should suggest that, when a drink of water has been either retained or vomited, a sweet drink such as diluted fruit juice or cordial should be given. It may be explained that the sweet drink prevents the child feeling sick as a result of a period of starvation. If this drink is vomited, suggest trying again shortly. When a drink is retained, soft food may be given. The essential message to be conveyed is that in moderate vomiting one should keep trying fluids. If the vomiting persists a doctor should be consulted in case the child has some intercurrent illness of which the vomiting is a symptom. The basis of this is that moderate vomiting after general anaesthesia is not uncommon and is harmless. Danger lies firstly in failing to recognize an intercurrent illness which may be serious, and less commonly, in the adverse metabolic effects of prolonged emesis.

CIRCULATORY ARREST

Although not common, circulatory arrest is a recognized complication of general anaesthesia. The emergency management of the condition by intermittent positive pressure breathing and closed chest cardiac massage is now well established and is widely taught. For circulatory arrest occurring in the course of general anaesthesia in hospital, with all facilities and skilled staff on hand, a salvage rate better than 25 per cent is usual. If the arrest occurs in the course of a general anaesthetic for a dental procedure management may present problems for several reasons. A plan of action such as is recommended for general surgical operating theatres (e.g., Gilston and Resnekov 1971) may need some modification. The anaesthetist will most likely be the only medical person present, it will be appropriate for him to take charge and direct resuscitation. He may need to take an electrocardiograph, insert an intravenous cannula and administer drugs. It will probably be necessary for him to delegate to a nurse the task of intermittent positive pressure ventilation of the patient. In this situation therefore, if there is not an endotracheal tube already in place, one should be inserted immediately. An untrained dental nurse who has been taught what to do may be capable of squeezing a bag, but not of simultaneously applying a face mask and maintaining a clear airway consistently.

If each person present is trained in performance of external heart massage and pulmonary ventilation, the management of the immediate emergency is relatively straightforward; unless there is very quick restoration of a normal heart beat, however, further definitive action is urgently required. This is a situation in anticipation of which planning is most necessary. The anaesthetist who administers general anaesthesia in a dental surgeon's rooms is well advised to study the problem of where to transfer a patient with a circulatory collapse and to decide in advance the soundest course of management in discussion with the staff of the nearest hospital. Following institution of artificial respiration and circulation, immediate steps should be taken to move the patient to the nearest appropriately equipped hospital, maintaining intermittent positive pressure ventilation with oxygen and, if indicated, uninterrupted external heart massage. Unless an arrest occurs actually in a hospital which is extremely well equipped in regard to cardiac monitoring and intensive care facilities the patient should be transferred early to such a hospital. How early this should be is a matter for judgment by an anaesthetist. It is easier and safer to transfer the patient after re-establishment of spontaneous heart action, but transfer should rarely be delayed for long in anticipation of this event.

CIRCULATORY COLLAPSE IN THE DENTAL SURGERY

Circulatory collapse may occur quite apart from general anaesthesia. The common collapse seen in the dental surgery is fainting—it is desirable that this be quickly recognized and correctly treated. Various ways are described of managing fainting, these include some which indicate a lack of understanding of the problem. There is a need to comprehend the apparent effectiveness of traditional treatments as well as the reasons for discarding them in favour of an alternative.

Fainting

Fainting is essentially a severe circulatory collapse with extreme fall of blood pressure and usually slowing of the heart rate. There is intense pallor of the skin—to the onlooker it can be most alarming, because the patient can momentarily appear to be dead. Provided that the patient is quickly placed, or allowed to fall, so that the head is not higher than the feet, recovery is invariable and quick. The point can hardly be over stressed that quick recovery is the diagnostic feature of fainting. Failure of recovery in spite of adequate treatment may be the only early sign that the diagnosis of fainting is incorrect: that one is in fact dealing with established circulatory arrest. In a case where 'treatment' to this point has consisted of 'smelling salts' under the nose, and especially where the patient is not supine but bent forward with the head between the knees, a complete change of attitude and procedure is necessary, and the essential treatment of circulatory arrest is irrevocably delayed.

'Smelling salts' used in fainting is merely a source of ammonia gas: if a patient breathes even slightly this provides an intensely painful stimulus. Any patient who is not in deep coma will respond by movement and by taking a breath, to the gratification of the person applying the stimulus; pulling the hair is as effective and less harmful. Instead of these one may apply measures to free the airway: lifting the jaw forward and sweeping a finger across the pharynx. These supply an equally effective stimulus which will indicate the occurrence of recovery. The advantage of using these measures is obvious: in the very rare event of a failure of recovery demonstrating the occurrence of circulatory arrest, treatment will be well advanced by the time the diagnosis is made.

A logical plan of treatment for fainting, therefore, is to apply invariably and immediately the early measures for management of circulatory arrest, until by recovery of consciousness the patient tells one to desist. Only in this way can dentists be brought to regard fainting with equanimity. It is important to have a sympathetic appreciation of the psychic trauma to the onlooker resulting from a sudden severe faint: this chiefly stems from a momentary, but intense fear that one is in fact witnessing a fatal collapse. When all staff are taught to treat every faint along these lines the improvement in morale is noticeable. A practical point which will be observed by the doctor in the dental clinic is a diminution in the number of urgent calls to attend people who have collapsed. No longer may he almost expect to arrive on the scene to find a completely recovered patient: he is now likely to be called only when there has been some failure of response to adequate treatment.

RARE COMPLICATIONS

To deal in detail with these may tend to create a false emphasis, but patients undergoing general anaesthesia for dental surgery may still be at risk from them. Malignant hyperpyrexia (Denborough *et al* 1962) is one such complication: a condition characterized by muscular rigidity and cyanosis with a rapidly fatal, extreme elevation of body temperature, the tendency to the development of the condition being, as a rule, strongly familial. It is dealt with to give an example of important points relative to any rare condition. A careful history may give warning, but it may not be the formal medical history. Fears and misgivings expressed to a nurse or other staff member by the patient or by a relative may give the only clue to the fact that there is a familial history of trouble with anaesthesia. Staff should be encouraged to pass on such information. In regard to recognizing the developing condition, the first necessity is to be aware of the possibility. After that it is a matter of monitoring the progress of the anaesthetic, and this term is used in its widest sense: not the mere setting and observing of circulatory monitors, but noting details, whether the degree of muscular relaxation matches that expected from the drugs administered, and whether the patient's colour is good. If a patient appears even slightly cyanosed, the careful anaesthetist will never merely increase the oxygen flow—he will check every detail of the patient's condition to find the cause. If he finds cyanosis and undue muscular tone, this may be the only clue to the occurrence of a potentially disastrous complication. The educated vigilance which enables a practitioner to recognize as significant small variations from a normal response, cannot be learned from books. It is a by-product of a meticulous, careful technique developed by sound training, self criticism, and practice in an environment where at least some of the time his work is subject to critical appraisal by other practitioners.

The problem of providing the Dental Undergraduate with balanced teaching on this type of complication is a vexed one. If some rare complications are given special mention, e.g. sickle-cell anaemia and porphyria, it is difficult to convey any idea of how many others there are besides. At the Royal Dental Hospital the matter is easier to manage because anaesthetic registrars receive clinical teaching in the same environment as the dental undergraduate performs some of his clinical work. As has already been mentioned in relation to management of common airway problems, the undergraduate inevitably receives a more balanced teaching in these circumstances than can be achieved by the most carefully prepared lecture course.

Complications of sedation

The point deserves emphasis, that sedation procedures which involve administration of agents capable of producing general anaesthesia have the potential for similar complications. The selection of patients and the manner of use of the procedure means that the complication rate will usually be very low, but will never be non-existent. The special problem of complications in relation to sedation procedures is examined in depth in Chapter 10.

CHAPTER 6
CLINICAL APPLICATION

This text began by setting out certain ideals in relation to general anaesthesia. In this chapter consideration is given to the compromise necessary in the application of these ideals to the dental out-patient clinic. A brief resumé is first made of some important points before dealing with details.

The anaesthetist should be a physician with special training: In the Dental School Clinic this is most important. Perhaps the dentist has in the past performed more efficiently in this field than the specialist anaesthetist: this shows up the need for the anaesthetist to understand the problem and to manage it better. Teaching of anaesthetists should be carried out in the Dental Clinic, where most basic skills of anaesthesia can be so readily practised and taught. Dentists need to learn about general anaesthesia at first hand—not necessarily to become skilled in its practice but to understand it and gain the background skills necessary for safe use of sedation procedures. For this they need a specialist anaesthetist as teacher.

The anaesthetist is to make a sufficient examination of the patient to determine his fitness: The importance of this has been minimized in Dental School teaching with the suggestion that the history and the appearance of the patient constitute an adequate guide to fitness for a dental anaesthetic. The role of the anaesthetist as physician in this context needs emphasis if teaching is to be sound.

The anaesthetist needs to have a sufficient knowledge of the surgery intended: This has received emphasis in relation to choice of anaesthetic technique and will be further stressed in relation to management of problem cases.

Post-operative management: This does not loom large in this context. Important points are that patients should be under observation for a sufficient period and that post-operative briefing should be soundly based.

When clinic organization is considered it will be with the objective of describing the implementation of a practice which, while being feasible and realistic is as close as possible to ideal in all respects. Clinical teaching can be sound only if day to day practice can be confidently pointed to as an example.

ORGANIZATION

The General Anaesthetic Clinic is a busy area in most Dental Schools: if it is to run smoothly and to be efficient sound organization is needed. Part of this is the delegation by professional staff to nursing and clerical staff of many matters of routine. The dentist and anaesthetist need to be well aware that this occurs, and that it is kept within bounds. If any departure from routine necessitates making a decision about patient management, this is the prerogative of the professional staff and must be referred to them. A weakness of the classical dental school practice was the attempt to deal with all cases with the same anaesthetic technique. Introduction of variety into techniques is a part only of the remedy: patient selection and management has often been equally stereotyped. The anaesthetist can make a contribution by learning something of dental surgery and the realistic problems of its performance. He also needs to be sure that pre-anaesthetic assessment of patients' medical condition is adequate, efficiently performed and soundly based.

Medical assessment of patients

When patients are to be admitted to hospital for abdominal or similar major surgery, examination in a pre-anaesthetic clinic is most valuable. It has been suggested therefore, that a similar routine be introduced in the dental school so that any patients booked for the general anaesthetic clinic can first be examined to determine their suitability for general anaesthesia. This is not altogether sound. The youth and good health of the majority of the patients, and the nature of the surgery, make it unrewarding.

Patients for major surgery are, on average, older than dental cases. There will be among them an appreciable incidence of significant pulmonary and cardiovascular disease. The detection, investigation and treatment of this prior to admission to hospital may be expected to confer tangible benefit in increased freedom from intra-operative and post-anaesthetic problems, as well as avoiding much of the inconvenience and wasted time resulting from late cancellation of operations due to the causes mentioned.

In dental cases these considerations are not applicable to the same extent. The number of cases is great—because of their youth and of selection by dental staff, the incidence of disease may be very low. Detection of significant disease usually means consideration of an alternative such as local analgesia: it would seldom lead to investigation and treatment to prepare the patient for general anaesthesia. The nature of the procedures is such that the occasional late cancellation will not seriously upset routine. There is little incentive for an anaesthetist to be thorough and efficient in performing routine examination of unselected dental cases prior to booking for general anaesthesia: there is an obvious need to seek a more realistic alternative, yet one conducive to soundness in teaching. One method that has been used in some clinics is that a medical questionnaire replaces the medical examination. There are clinics in which a questionnaire constitutes the only medical assessment, it is signed by the patient and is held as a document which would defend the dentist against allegations of negligence should the patient prove to be not healthy. It is felt that this is a misuse of a technique which can be a valuable adjunct to medical examination.

Medical assessment of patients is sometimes attempted in another way. The dentist—or an auxiliary—may measure certain clinical parameters, e.g. pulse rate and blood pressure, or—especially on the North American continent—a number of biochemical tests and perhaps an electrocardiograph are taken for the consideration of the dentist in making a clinical assessment of the patient. This rather ignores the important point that in taking a medical history and making a pre-anaesthetic examination of a patient, the anaesthetist is a physician making a diagnosis of the patient's condition as a basis for decisions about general anaesthesia.

Screening of patients

If the anaesthetist can be asked to see in advance of booking only a smaller number of patients, those who have been selected for the reason that their health is suspect, he will find this task more rewarding and will provide a more effective consultative service in every way than is possible if he is beseiged by large numbers of healthy patients.

As decisions by dentists about patient management should be made only after some enquiry into their general medical condition, current practice is that a questionnaire is filled in by all patients undergoing dental examination and treatment at the Royal Dental Hospital. It was developed originally as a pre-anaesthetic assessment but has been extended and modified to cover most aspects of general health relevant to dental treatment (Fig. 27). It is so phrased that questions are answered 'yes' or 'no', and so designed that negative answers suggest that the patient is healthy, affirmative answers suggest the need for further investigation. Each patient is requested to fill in the questionnaire before seeing the professional staff, assistance being given by a nurse or clerk, or an interpreter if needed. The fact of having the questions put begins the patient's anamnesis and facilitates subsequent history taking.

Questions to which 'yes' is the answer should be followed up by the examining dentist, who tries to determine whether there is significant evidence of ill-health, and he may refer the patient for medical consultation if he feels that this is indicated. The patient who is thus referred is already thinking about his past medical history and current therapy, and the positive features of any illness are noted on the questionnaire. It is easy, in these circumstances, to elicit a satisfactory history fairly quickly. Because of the relatively small number of patients selected in this way, medical history and examination can take a little time, and be thoroughly carried out. In this way a sound basis can be established for decisions about patient management.

One can hardly over-emphasize the importance, when cases are referred for consultation, of taking an adequate history and making a careful examination and a considered diagnosis. Too often the pre-anaesthetic assessment of dental patients has been described as wholly centred about estimation of the patient's exercise tolerance, as if to imply that 'the patient who can stand up to exercise can stand the strain of a general anaesthetic'. The question of the diagnostic significance of patients' varying exercise tolerance is ignored. Such teaching can only tend to convey to dental undergraduate and graduate students the false idea that there is little to the practice of medicine and general anaesthesia. They are apt to gain the impression, for example, that auscultation of the heart prior to administration of a

Form 114

THE ROYAL DENTAL HOSPITAL OF MELBOURNE

QUESTIONS CONCERNING GENERAL HEALTH

Hospital Code	Card Type	Unit No.	Date of Birth	Treatment Date
A 1 1				

NAME: ....

Please answer all the questions —

    If your answer is **YES** to the question, put a circle around YES

    If your answer is **NO** to the question, put a circle around NO

    All questions to be answered by, or on behalf of the patient.

1.	Are you being treated for any condition by a physician now?	YES	NO
2.	Are you taking any drugs or medicines now? Or in the last six months.	YES	NO
3.	Have you ever had any of the following : —		
	Heart Trouble	YES	NO
	Rheumatic Fever	YES	NO
	High Blood Pressure	YES	NO
	Jaundice or Hepatitis	YES	NO
	Stroke	YES	NO
	Diabetes	YES	NO
	Asthma	YES	NO
	Persistent Cough	YES	NO
	Chest Trouble	YES	NO
	Fits or Epilepsy	YES	NO
	Heart Murmur	YES	NO
4.	Have you ever had any other long or serious illness?	YES	NO
5.	Have you ever had a bad reaction to any of the following : —		
	Aspirin	YES	NO
	Penicillin	YES	NO
	Any other drugs, medicines or injections	YES	NO
6.	Have you ever had serious bleeding needing special treatment?	YES	NO
7.	Have you ever had a bad reaction to —		
	Dental Treatment	YES	NO
	General Anaesthetic	YES	NO
8.	**Females:** If pregnant, please write here / /19		
	showing due date		

Signed: ....
    Patient
    Parent
    Guardian
        Date: ....

Comment by Professional Staff:

Fig. 27. In assessment of a patient's general health, questions should be about factual history rather than about symptoms.

general anaesthetic is performed solely for the detection of 'murmurs' which might constitute an indication for 'antibiotic cover' but which have no other significance. This type of practice has regrettably been a contributing factor to the tendency for dental undergraduates to gain a sketchy, empirical knowledge of medicine: this position can be remedied most effectively by having dental students and graduates in frequent contact with sound medical practice in relation to their own patients. The student should be regularly able to see a sound clinical exposition and demonstration, in which the history and clinical findings of his patient are integrated by a thoughtful physician to lead to a considered diagnosis. In this way he may be able to gain an adequate notion of what is involved in the practice of medicine.

In the teaching hospital and in private practice the anaesthetist is apt to be the medical practitioner with whom the dentist has closest contact, the doctor whom he sees at work. If he sees always hasty, cursory examinations, a few brief leading questions and a guess-work assessment, then his opinion of medical practice will be low, his respect for its practitioners will diminish, he will be unable to make best use of consultation with his patient's doctor.

Anaesthetists need to make an effort to get out of the bad habits of cursory patient assessment into which they have sometimes been pushed by the sheer weight of numbers of patients presenting in the practice of out-patient dental anaesthesia. An appropriate organization can be developed so that it is easy to manage patients correctly.

Selection of patients

The dentist who examines patients and refers them for, among other procedures, extraction of teeth, needs to know something of the indications for general anaesthesia. Whether such indications can or should be laid down dogmatically is open to question. It is possible to perform most dental procedures under local analgesia: the risk to life of such a procedure is virtually nil. Administration of a general anaesthetic always involves a risk to life although the risk may be quite small (Speirs 1953).

It is usual in such texts as this to set out a list of 'Indications for General Anaesthesia'. As a rule this comprises those groups of cases in which, in the Author's opinion, the use of local analgesia is not feasible whether because of idiosyncrasy, infection, lack of co-opera-tion or magnitude of surgery. It is useful sometimes to have such a list to guide one's thoughts on this subject when making decisions about patient management. It is most undesirable, however, that such a decision should ever be made on a basis of empiricism. Caution needs to be exercised in particular in relation to acceptance of patients' statements about adverse reactions to local anaesthesia as an indication for general anaesthesia. The following cases may serve to illustrate this point.

Case 1: A middle-aged man requiring extraction of some teeth was referred for consideration of general anaesthesia because of a previous 'bad reaction to local anaesthetic'. Careful questioning revealed that some years before, following extraction of a left lower tooth with local anaesthetic injection, he had suffered a few hours later with severe frontal headache, nausea and vomiting, drooping of the left eyelid and paralysis of the ocular muscles with double vision—necessitating his admission to hospital. This history suggested that the symptoms arose from an intracranial aneurysm and this was the diagnosis which had, in fact, been made on his admission to hospital. The timing of events indicated that any causal relation with local anaesthetic injection was most unlikely. The decision was made that general anaesthesia should be avoided, and he was treated uneventfully with local analgesia.

Case 2: A male aged 70 gave a history of 'adverse reaction to local' in that an extraction under local anaesthetic had been followed by a rash and severe eye trouble on the same side as the injection. Detailed history revealed that he had attended his dentist with severe pain in the upper jaw: local anaesthetic was injected and an upper tooth extracted. The extraction did not hurt but the original pain persisted and next day a vesicular rash developed about the cheek and eye on the same side and this was followed by corneal ulceration. This history, and the scarring which was faintly visible suggested that the condition was herpes zoster rather than reaction to local anaesthetic.

To return then to the dentist who selects general anaesthesia for a patient who is to have extraction of teeth. This decision is in a measure tentative pending examination of the patient by the anaesthetist. The plan will seldom be changed, however: it is therefore most desirable that the initial decision of the dentist for general anaesthesia in preference to local be soundly based. This is most likely to occur if the dentist has had experience of working with sound general anaesthesia in conditions such as those already described. There are advantages in dental students—graduate and undergraduate—working in the clinic while anaesthetic registrars are learning the practice of dental anaesthesia. No attempt need be made to minimize incidents or difficulties: these, and the active measures to deal with them can be realistically discussed and demonstrated. Anaesthetic registrars will be medical men who have made anaesthesia their special study and practice for some time. The dentist will see that they still have their difficulties and he will readily gain an appreciation of the problems of general anaesthesia as well as its potential. He may be expected as a result of such experience not only to make sound decisions in the case of healthy patients but also to be ready to seek consultation with the anaesthetist about any patient whose medical condition is in question. The development of this attitude will have benefits which go far beyond selection of patients for general anaesthetic and will be a means of ensuring that dental staff and students gain a deeper appreciation of the discipline of medicine than has sometimes been the case. The emphasis in teaching clinical medicine to dental undergraduates has been placed on development of a facility for 'spot diagnosis': medicine has been learned, as it were from the Clinical Picture Book. The dentist can hardly fail to increase his appreciation of medicine when his essays at diagnosis are readily put to the touchstone of enlightened medical practice.

Briefing of patients

When general anaesthesia is administered to out-patients it is necessary for safety that instructions be conveyed effectively to patients to ensure their observance of essential prerequisites. It is most desirable to have a printed list of instructions the wording of which is carefully planned (Figs. 28 and 29). At the time when the booking is made for the procedure, the patient or parent should also be given the important instructions verbally as well as being asked to sign the slip. This signature acknowledges the instructions as well as giving permission for administration of a general anaesthetic. For out-patients the signature is not witnessed. Most of the patients are minors: the parent is usually present: the implied consent of bringing the patient as arranged is perhaps of more value than the doubtful formality of a second signature on a form.

A problem relating to consent for general anaesthesia, which is being increasingly encountered, is one related to greater freedom and mobility of young people at an early age. This is the consent for treatment of the young person who is under the legal age of attainment of majority, but is living an independent existence away from his parents. The error to be avoided here is that clerical staff may

Form 8

The Royal Dental Hospital of Melbourne
711 Elizabeth Street, Melbourne, 3000
Telephone: 347 4222

Patients attending for treatment under General Anaesthetic or Sedation must follow these instructions.

REPORT TO:... Phone: 347 4222
(Telephone this extension if unable to attend) Ext.............

DATE:...

TIME:...

On this day:—

1. **NO FOOD OR DRINK** may be taken from midnight before attendance.
2. The patient **MUST BE ACCOMPANIED** by a responsible adult, who will arrange transport and care for the patient.
3. The patient **MUST NOT DRIVE A CAR**, travel alone or engage in responsible work for 8 hours after the procedure.
4. Children **MUST BE WATCHED** to see that they do not eat or drink : they must not go to school that day.
5. Teeth must be cleaned before attending.

PATIENT

NAME:.. AGE: ....

REG. No...

ADDRESS: ....

I have read and followed the above instructions.

I consent to the administration of a General Anaesthetic
to —
* The abovenamed patient.
* Myself.

SIGNED..
* Patient
* Parent
* Guardian
* Cross out which is inapplicable.

**Bring this form with you when you attend. It must be signed.
You must notify the Hospital if unable to keep this appointment —
otherwise re-booking may be refused.**

Fig. 28. Briefing slip for morning general anaesthetic. The signature of patient or parent on the slip acknowledges the instructions and gives permission for anaesthetic.

The Royal Dental Hospital of Melbourne

711 Elizabeth Street, Melbourne, 3000
Telephone: 347 4222

Patients attending for treatment under General Anaesthetic or Sedation must follow these instructions.

REPORT TO:.. Phone: 347 4222
(Telephone this extension if unable to attend) Ext..............

DATE:..

TIME:..

On this day:—

1. **A LIGHT BREAKFAST** to be eaten not later than **7.30 a.m.: it should be tea or fruit juice with bread or toast — NO milk, meat or eggs. NOTHING to eat or drink after that.**
2. The patient **MUST BE ACCOMPANIED** by a responsible adult, who will arrange transport and care for the patient.
3. The patient **MUST NOT DRIVE A CAR,** travel alone or engage in responsible work for 8 hours after the procedure.
4. Children **MUST BE WATCHED** to see that they do not eat or drink : they must not go to school that day.
5. Teeth must be cleaned before attending.

PATIENT

NAME:... AGE:...........

REG. No. ....

ADDRESS:...

I have read and followed the above instructions.
I consent to the administration of a General Anaesthetic
to —
    * The abovenamed patient.
    * Myself.

                                        * Patient
SIGNED... * Parent
                                        * Guardian
        * Cross out which is inapplicable.

**Bring this form with you when you attend. It must be signed.
You must notify the Hospital if unable to keep this appointment —
otherwise re-booking may be refused.**

Fig. 29.   Briefing slip for afternoon general anaesthetic. Instructions about eating and fasting need to be detailed and definite.

readily accept the word of the patient that he is living independently of his parents, and have such a minor sign his own permission for general anaesthesia. Alternatively if such a patient is accompanied by an adult, an attempt is sometimes made to have this adult acquaintance sign permission for anaesthesia. Unless the person is in fact the guardian of the minor, this is not acceptable: it is unreasonable to press a mere acquaintance of a patient to sign such a document. This person may be of assistance in another way, if he is aware of the patient's circumstances and is able to state definitely that the patient does in fact live independently apart from his parents. A signed statement to this effect is of significant value in backing up a decision to accept, as permission for general anaesthesia, the signature of a minor. All responsible staff need to have a clear idea of what they are doing to avoid problems in this field. It is wise however to refer such cases to a senior professional man, preferably the anaesthetist, who should take a history and examine the patient as well as discussing his circumstances. Such an examination will occasionally reveal most significant findings—a somewhat disturbed girl was found to be suffering from malnutrition and chronic respiratory infection, an eighteen year old proved to be in an advanced stage of pregnancy and denied all knowledge of it. Such cases should of course be sorted out before proceeding to extraction of teeth with general anaesthesia. Most often the patient is healthy and reasonable, and is requested to write to his parents and obtain their written consent for general anaesthesia and dental treatment. There are two important desiderata—to satisfy oneself that the procedure is reasonable, and to have, in the patient's record, a satisfactory signed permission.

Reception

Reception and handling of patients in a busy clinic needs to be on a sound but simple system if errors of identity and the like are to be avoided, and problems recognized and dealt with. Booking for surgery under general anaesthetic is the first stage of reception: for this to be done the patient needs to present with a recommendation signed by a staff dentist that surgery be performed with general anaesthesia. He also needs to have a medical questionnaire completed, and signed by the examining dentist. On sighting these the clerk makes the appointment, and issues the appropriate briefing slip according to the time of appointment: she should reiterate the instructions and ensure that there is available someone who can take the responsibility of signing the form. The history comprising examination sheet and questionnaire remains in the clinic, the briefing slip goes with the patient to be brought back on the day of the procedure.

On this day the clerk matches the patient with the history, checks that the briefing slip is signed, asks about fasting and any recent illness—e.g. a cold in the head. She weighs the patient and records the weight in kilograms on the history. Then she attaches an identifying band on the left wrist of the patient. This has on it, in addition to registered number and name, a note to show who accompanies the patient—e.g. **MUM** or **DAD**—which assists recovery staff in calling parents when the patient wakes up, or the dentist or anaesthetist who needs to consult the parent on any point.

The anaesthetist can see on the examination sheet the scope of surgery intended and age and weight of patient. He sees on the medical sheet a note of any problems and some elucidation of them. He checks the name on the wrist band, makes such examination as seems to be indicated, and is ready to proceed with the anaesthetic by the most appropriate technique.

THE NON-FASTING PATIENT

Despite careful briefing, patients sometimes attend having taken food when they should be fasting. Clerical and nursing staff become expert in the detection of these breaches. If they find that food or drink has been taken, they should refer the patient to the anaesthetist for a decision on what to do. This is an important decision—it should not be delegated, nor should it be made as a rule without seeing the patient. There is a conflict here which needs to be resolved. The views on fasting in preparation for general anaesthesia which are set out in many text books on dental anaesthesia tend to be unduly narrow and empirical in saying that fasting is mandatory. In contrast to this, the readiness with which an experienced consultant will give an anaesthetic to a non-fasting patient may quite perplex the conscientious dental undergraduate. It is most desirable that a consistent basis be established for these decisions so that they may be sound and comprehensible. The objective is plain—to do what is best for the patient in the circumstances which obtain. If a patient has not fasted the professional staff should quietly accept matters as they are, consider all aspects of the situation and try to arrive at a sound decision.

The anaesthetist needs to guard against too ready a delegation of authority in this sphere. Even in the middle of a busy list, if a clerk or nurse asks for example: "we have a four-year-old who had a drink of milk at 7 a.m. Will we put her at the end of the list?", the reply should be: "I shall have to look at the patient".

The examination may be of the briefest, but it is essential that it be carried out if one is to avoid sometimes being put in an invidious position. If the patient happens to have, for example, a receding jaw and limited mouth opening which could make dealing with vomiting a matter of extreme difficulty, one could have cause to regret a casual decision to proceed, made without seeing the patient.

A rigid, unbending, ritualistic enforcement of a rule of fasting with no exceptions may not achieve its objective. It may tend merely to encourage concealment and prevarication among patients. It is better to aim for a high rate of fasting, and to try to ensure that, when one is dealing with a non-fasting patient, the fact is clearly known to all concerned so that the case will be handled carefully and expeditiously, and that all emergency equipment will be ready for immediate use.

Of the various aspects which need to be taken into account, food in the stomach is only one. Its presence may contribute to the risk of vomiting and aspiration, but other factors are also significant (see Chapter 5, p. 63). Anything which militates against smooth anaesthesia should be sought after. If it is observed for example that a patient has a respiratory infection which may give rise to trouble from coughing and laryngospasm, this would be a point in favour of postponement to another day. On the other hand, it may appear that a child who has taken some food has a neglected appearance, one may feel on this account that the chance of the child being genuinely fasted on a future occasion may be remote. It may be preferable to take a predictable risk immediately rather than an unknown risk at a later date.

The question of whether the operation is urgent or not also needs consideration. Although there is generally no risk to life from dental conditions, they may be very painful. When a question of dental urgency arises the dentist also should examine the patient, in an attempt to assess what is the degree of surgical urgency—the two practitioners then have a sound basis on which to make a decision.

PATIENTS WITH 'COLDS'

A common problem in anaesthesia and surgery is the patient who presents for general anaesthesia, but is suffering from symptoms suggesting respiratory tract infection. This problem bedevils anaesthetist and surgeon wherever they work and it is sometimes dealt with on a basis of extreme empiricism. An anaesthetist will frequently make decisions on this problem, but may have little opportunity to follow up the postponed cases, to know whether his decision was justified. Most anaesthetists know little of what may be the ill effects of the mere administration of a general anaesthetic to a patient with respiratory infection. Obviously, the patient who has some degree of bronchitis will be at special risk following upper abdominal surgery under general anaesthesia, the risks will be of bronchial obstruction and its sequelae. In the context of dental anaesthesia the concern is more for the immediate influence of respiratory infections on conduct of a short general anaesthetic. The Dental Out-patient Clinic offers a unique field of practice in this matter. Opportunities are provided for an anaesthetist to find out, at first hand, some of the problems associated with general anaesthesia in the presence of respiratory infection.

The principles already noted relative to fasting apply here. Any evidence of a cold or cough should be assiduously sought by all staff. If any is found, the patient should be examined by the anaesthetist and a decision made. One needs to make a diagnosis on the basis of findings, concerning both the patient's general health and the intercurrent illness. The history of the cold is important. How long have symptoms been present, when did they start? Has nasal discharge remained watery or become purulent? Has there been a cough? For how long? What treatment has been given? It is important to determine whether the current symptoms represent, for example, the final stage of a mild infection, or the early stage of a severe infection. Examination will include at least auscultation of heart and chest and looking at the nose and throat—taking the temperature may be a valuable adjunct. Experience shows that in case of complaint of sore throat, examination may reveal anything from a normal throat to acute membranous tonsillitis—it is most necessary to look.

On the basis that the cold is in its closing stages one may proceed with an anaesthetic—perhaps for the relief of acute dental pain. It is sometimes found that there is extreme irritability and over-responsiveness of the laryngeal reflex, which makes maintenance of smooth anaesthesia difficult. On other occasions there may be no difficulty of this sort in such a case. It is difficult to tell which is the case which is likely to give trouble. A clinical sign which may be of value is the response of the child on taking several deep breaths. A paroxysm of coughing, especially if there are any moist sounds heard in the chest, strongly suggests that smooth induction of anaesthesia may be difficult. Many details concerning the effects of minor respiratory infection on the course of general anaesthesia emerge from this type of practice. The trainee anaesthetist, working under supervision, can gain first hand experience of some value in giving him a sound basis for this difficult type of decision in all fields of anaesthetic practice.

Premedication

As a prelude to out-patient general anaesthesia, premedication so increases the risks and difficulties, for so little benefit, that it is virtually never used: the rare occasion on which it is felt to be necessary should be made a special occasion, and the patient is better treated as an in-patient, or at least as a day patient. With reasonably gentle, confident handling and a skilful intravenous induction, premedication is unnecessary. If a patient is to be intubated, some atropine may be given with the induction dose of intravenous agent, it is generally omitted with non-endotracheal anaesthetics.

RECOVERY

This is one of the most testing areas of the whole organization, and is sometimes not well handled. It is vitally necessary that it be closely supervised by a competent general trained nurse, versed in the skills of airway care and emergency treatment. It is also desirable that all anaesthetists take an active and sympathetic interest in the problems of the recovery room.

The nurse in charge of recovery should be well trained and confident. A person who is not familiar with caring for unconscious patients will never be happy unless the patient is exhibiting signs of activity, in which case patients will not be allowed to recover quietly but will be stimulated, shouted at and shaken into responsiveness. The policy which should be clearly defined is that patients shall be observed and allowed to wake spontaneously. There is apt to be maintained a pretence that anaesthesia is being practised on an ambulatory basis, that the patient should be ready to walk out of the theatre. If this is so, then the unfortunate patient may be sponged with ice cold water and stimulated by pinching, slapping and shouting while still in the chair: these practices are intolerable, and need to be discouraged.

The recovering patient should be recumbent in the 'post-tonsil-lectomy' position to sleep off his anaesthetic under the supervision of a nurse. In this way a high proportion of quiet recoveries may be achieved. Recovery will not always be smooth and quiet, however. The staff need to be able to handle any situation, including the restless frightened child who is screaming and is also bleeding from all quadrants of the mouth. This can be learned only by experience, but a few comments are made relative to the problems of teaching in this field.

First, and most important, the anaesthetist in charge needs to be thoroughly well versed and skilful in this testing and rather menial task, and be able and willing to teach it. The ability to handle such a situation is a skill well worth having, it is, unfortunately, not easy to obtain such practical experience during training, and this applies equally to nurses, to medical undergraduates, and to anaesthetic registrars.

The recovery room of the large Teaching Hospital tends, to an increasing extent, to a less rapid turnover of patients, and to place more emphasis on 'post-surgical' management, with less on post-anaesthetic. The trainee nurse who attends recovery room may learn little but management of chest and bladder drains, continuous wash-outs, and monitoring of central venous pressure and electrocardio-graph. Simple airway problems seem to receive little attention, they are not, as a rule, permitted to interfere with the teaching of post-surgical management, they are no longer the very stuff of which recovery room teaching is made.

In a busy surgical hospital, tremendous reliance is placed upon the trained nurse in charge of Recovery Room, in regard to her capabilities at airway maintenance in the patient recovering from general anaesthesia. If her experience has been gained in surroundings such as those just outlined as characterizing the recovery room of a large Teaching Hospital then her practical experience in the vital areas of her training may be relatively slight.

The post-anaesthetic recovery room of the Out-patient Dental Theatre offers opportunities almost without parallel for repetitive experience in management of recovery in circumstances which invite the occurrence of minor airway difficulties. Nurses and doctors alike can benefit from this concentrated experience, of repeated practical instruction in aspiration of mouth and pharynx, of recognizing and dealing with minor airway spasms, of arrest of haemorrhage in the mouth. It is for this reason that the following points of detail relative to the management of the recovery situation are included.

It is advisable to stand behind the patient, leaning over him. His top shoulder and arm can be held back with the right elbow and the forehead held with the left forearm, to extend the neck, leaving both hands free to manipulate sucker and packs (Fig. 30). One aspirates the dependent cheek first (Fig. 31), this will clear most of the blood and indicate level of consciousness. A purposive response to this indicates a very light plane of unconsciousness.

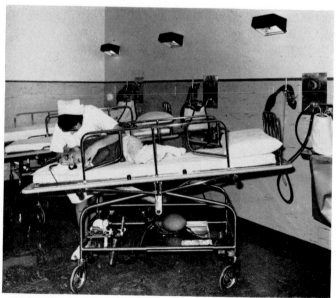

Fig. 30. The nurse has more control of the situation when behind the patient. She is not forced to 'dodge' if the patient coughs.

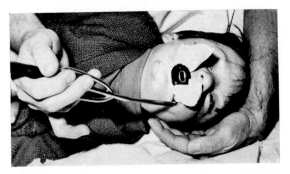

Fig. 31.   Blood tends to pool in the cheek on the side which is dependent
and may be readily sucked out from there.

An attempt should be made to look in the mouth to see if there is
blood or clot within the arch of the teeth. If there is, then it should be
sucked out. This is a task requiring expertise, and its safe achievement depends on recognition of certain principles governing patient
response. The patient is persuaded to open his jaws, the sucker is
inserted, the end of the sucker should be directed immediately to the
pharynx, close to the midline, remaining in contact with the dorsum
of the tongue. If there is no response the procedure is easy. but the
patient is deeply unconscious and needs watching. If, as is usual, there
is a response, it will be of gagging or retching, in process of which the
mouth opens widely (Fig. 32). This gives a moment or two of good
exposure, to inspect and aspirate the pharynx and to place fresh
packs over bleeding sockets as needed (Fig. 33) then to remove the

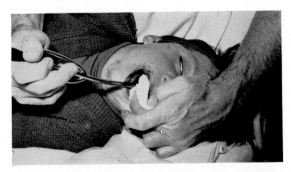

Fig. 32.   Insertion of the sucker handpiece into the pharynx in the recovering patient induces wide mouth opening and gives an opportunity to
change packs.

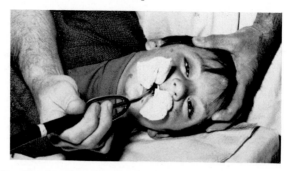

Fig. 33.   The insertion of packs should be completed before the mouth closes again.

sucker before the teeth clamp shut on it. The whole procedure must be quick, gentle and decisive.

When packs have been placed over bleeding sockets, it may be necessary to hold the mandible up to maintain the pressure necessary for haemostasis. Extreme restlessness occasionally results from this, one needs then to look for one or both of two factors. The pressure may be causing pain, and need to be redistributed or modified, or the grip may be causing suffocation, with its resultant extreme restlessness and fighting. Granting a free airway will immediately diminish the restlessness. It should be forbidden for parents or relatives to be present during this non-co-operative phase of recovery, which

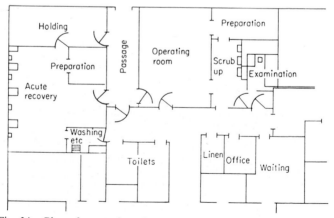

Fig. 34.   Plan of out-patient theatre area: note the examination room close to the theatre and a holding area adjacent to the acute recovery room.

should, if possible, be conducted in a sound-proofed area. It is inhumane to allow parents to see their children semi-conscious and bleeding, and the presence of even the best-behaved of parents may be a dangerously inhibiting factor in effective and safe management of the recovery.

Children should be held in the acute recovery area only long enough for significant haemorrhage to stop, and for the child to become reasonably conscious, aware, and—it is hoped—co-operative. For the remainder of their period of observation they can be with their parents, in the holding area.

HOLDING AREA

This is a room with seating or reclining accommodation for patients and their escorts, adjacent to but separate from the acute recovery area (Figs. 34 and 35). In any practice it is a desirable feature: in a teaching hospital it is vital. If the facility is available to retain patients for observation, then they will be observed, and trainee dentists and anaesthetists can learn, at first hand, the problems associated with

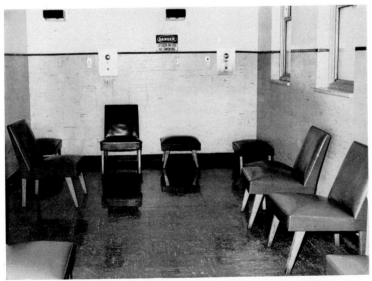

Fig. 35. The holding area has sitting or reclining accommodation for patients and their escorts.

recovery from anaesthesia and surgery. If patients are sent away too quickly a number of minor complications will be unseen and unknown, because their magnitude was not sufficient to necessitate return to hospital.

When a critical assessment is to be made of any technique of general anaesthesia or sedation, in relation to its use on an outpatient basis, it is essential that patients on whom it has been used be observed for some time after completion of the procedure. Such observation quickly modifies one's views on the suitability of intravenous diazepam, and even of methohexitone, as sedative agents for ambulatory out-patients. Following the use of either agent, patients who sit down to rest may very readily drop off to sleep.

Before patients are discharged, the mouth is inspected to ensure that active bleeding has ceased, and the patient will have been sitting and standing sufficiently to be sure that fainting or early vomiting is unlikely. A written briefing is desirable, covering the essential features most of which have already been dealt with, namely haemorrhage, vomiting, and, in the case of children who have been intubated, notes on recognition of and dealing with 'croup', suitable forms are reproduced in Fig. 36. If the nature of the clientele demand it, their translation into other languages should be effected.

STAFFING

When out-patient general anaesthesia is practised in the Dental School 'gas room' it has been usual for a general trained nurse to head the staff, and her responsibilities have sometimes spread over many areas. She has frequently been a king-pin in the organization, maintaining continuity and uniformity of practice as staff dentists come and go, and being in large measure responsible for drilling of dental students in the routine of the gas room. When general anaesthesia was taught and practised as an empirical, practical art, dentists would virtually learn anaesthesia from the sister in charge, in much the way that obstetric house surgeons learned from the experienced labour ward staff and the resident medical officer from his ward sister.

With the introduction to the Dental School of more modern teaching and practice of anaesthesia, the duties of the sister in charge become modified. She will be responsible for maintaining supplies of

INSTRUCTIONS FOR PATIENTS FOLLOWING
GENERAL ANAESTHESIA

fter returning home, the patient should rest.

leeding: If this persists or starts again -
                            Find the place which is bleeding.
                            Wipe away excess clot.
                            Place on the socket a large wad of cloth
                            covered material and have the patient bite
                            firmly on it for twenty minutes.

rinking and eating: The first drink should be plain water - it may
                            be vomited, with swallowed blood.
                            Sweet drinks should be taken next: cordial
                            or fruit juice with sugar and water.   (Milk is
                            not given at this stage.)
                            Small drinks should be taken repeatedly,
                            even if some are vomited.
                            Food may be taken when desired, it should be
                            soft and not too hot.

eek advice: If bleeding cannot be stopped by the measures
                            described.
                            If vomiting persists beyond four hours.
                            If any other matter causes concern.

Fig. 36.   Post-operative briefing for parents of child patients needs to
indicate clearly what to do and when to seek help.

SPECIAL INSTRUCTIONS FOLLOWING ENDOTRACHEAL ANAESTHETIC IN CHILDREN

NAME: REG. NO. :   DATE:

Your child had an anaesthetic given today by a tube in the windpipe. As this is very occasionally followed by some difficulty with breathing, please watch for the following, which may be warning signs:

Croup – this is a noisy, brassy cough which cause some distress. If it occurs, then watch the child and listen to its breathing when it is resting quietly and not crying. If breathing is persistently noisy or difficult, please have a doctor see the child and show him this form.

ANAESTHETIC DETAILS

DURATION: RELAXANT USED:

TIME OF INDUCTION: a. m.

                            p. m.

REMARKS:

equipment and drugs, and for supervising patient care, especially in the recovery room. When the modern anaesthetist deals with a series of cases, he is willing to delegate responsibility for care of the recovering patient in a nearby recovery room, but only if the person in charge is a general trained nurse. For induction of anaesthesia he will wish to have an assistant, but this can be a dental nurse or trainee, who needs merely to learn the few skills noted in Chapter 3. Following completion of induction she should continue to assist if the anaesthetic is non-endotracheal, or in any case, to provide necessary head support. The surgeon usually has two assistants, one to use the sucker and retractors at need, the other to pass packs and instruments. This can be reduced to one if the nurse is skilled, or in the teaching environment a dental student can fill one rôle. Two further nurses are desirable to assist in theatre and recovery. This may sound an extravagant staff, but when the theatre is busy the staff will all be hard pushed. Where a list of cases is to be done, the irreducible minimum is: a responsible person in recovery, a capable assistant for the anaesthetist and one for the surgeon, one circulating nurse to assist in recovery or theatre as needed. Numbers can be reduced further only if one accepts the delay inherent in the anaesthetist personally supervising the recovery of each patient. Where teaching is important the larger staff is mandatory.

PART III

SEDATION

Where general anaesthesia is a highly developed science and clinical discipline, medical anaesthetists are apt to decry the administration by dental practitioners of any general anaesthesia or sedation. Having seen the benefits especially in relation to major surgery on sick patients, of general anaesthesia being administered only under ideal conditions and by highly qualified specialists, they feel that every patient having an anaesthetic merits unselective application of the same high standards.

The use of sedation by dental practitioners however is well established in many parts of the world and will not be prevented by non-specific denunciation of the practice by a section of the medical profession. It is unrealistic to suggest that all such administrations should be performed by trained anaesthetists if only because of the prodigious numbers involved. The feasibility of training sufficient anaesthetists is questionable. More important, they would probably not be well motivated in routine performance of simple sedation procedures.

There is no easy solution to this problem. If any changes are to be made they should be initiated by involvement in these practices of the specialist anaesthetist. He must learn, at first hand, how to carry out sedation procedures and make over a period of time, a careful assessment of what is their place, scope and safety or otherwise in various hands.

This is, in fact, what has been attempted and the chapters which follow are based on experience in this field. Although a fairly thorough study of sedation procedures has been made, and they have been applied in many fields of surgery besides dental, the specialist anaesthetist does not become expert in the use of dental sedation in the way in which many dentists do. The specialist anaesthetist who practises in this field may have a small first-hand experience of the problems involved but, having applied the methods to patients in various categories of risk from medical and surgical disability he has, perhaps, a keener insight into their potential dangers.

The main objective is twofold: firstly to make these procedures comprehensible and credible to anaesthetists—for all too often the anaesthetist has failed badly in his attempts to emulate the 'Intravenous dentist' in particular. Secondly, because of his experience with a more varied group of patients and his background knowledge of medicine, the specialist anaesthetist becomes aware of potential sources of danger from these procedures. An attempt has been made to delineate these for they have too often been dismissed as nonexistent, or as easily avoidable by rigid adherence to a particular technique.

CHAPTER 7
DEFINITION AND BASIC CONCEPT

In relation to its use in dentistry, sedation has been defined as 'that state induced by a drug or drugs in which a patient remains conscious but is rendered less apprehensive. Protective reflexes are retained and the patient responds to an oral command. There may be a diminished sense of pain, but local analgesia may be required for some procedures. Partial or total amnesia may be experienced'. This definition implies that it is possible so to regulate the administration of drugs that there is only a moderate and predictable depression of consciousness. In fact, one of the hazards implicit in almost any sedation procedure is accidental progression to general anaesthesia. Safety, therefore, can only be partly assured by stipulations concerning which drugs should be used and how they should be given. There is no such thing as a 'safe' sedation procedure. The important consideration in this regard is what training and skill a dental practitioner should have for the safe administration of various types of sedation. An alternative would be what measure of supervision by a physician is needed for safety of the patient.

From time immemorial, sedation of one form or another has been used in preparation for various ordeals, but it has not always been admitted that the effect of the agent used was actually 'sedative'. Although it is in fact a cerebral depressant, alcohol in the form of a nip of spirits was highly regarded as a stimulant which strengthened and fortified one against various threats, of which dental treatment was one. A number of drugs have been self administered in preparation for a dental visit, varying with the culture to which the patient belongs and with his social standing, through barbiturate, chloral hydrate, and aspirin type analgesic to phenothiazines and benzodiazepines.

The supposed threat which dental treatment holds for the patient, who may therefore seek sedation, is twofold: pain and fear. The anticipation of pain or discomfort or of unpleasant effects from treatment is, of course, one of the sources of the fear or anxiety. There is also a fear, innate or acquired, which some persons exhibit towards having anything done to their teeth or mouth.

There has been a good deal written on the nature and causation of the intense fear which some people show relative to procedures in the mouth, based on explanations in terms of Freudian and other psychological theory. It is not intended to comment on the theory but merely to accept the clinical fact that these fears exist and to attempt to allay them by using the techniques of anaesthesia. It is necessary to recognize however, that psychotherapy, whether intentional or incidental, may profoundly influence the behaviour of the patient who is so afflicted, and that such psychotherapy may be sometimes facilitated by the effects of drugs administered for sedation.

LOCAL ANAESTHESIA

The painful nature of dental surgery has sometimes received consideration to the virtual exclusion of the other anxieties noted. Proponents of this approach tend to recommend the use of local analgesia, ignoring all other methods. Local analgesia has been a boon in dental treatment in that it can make the treatment painless, but it has very real limitations. The injection is usually unpleasant, if not actually painful, its administration may be followed by unpleasant subjective effects and even by fainting, its persistence of action beyond the time of treatment may cause discomfort and inconvenience, it may sometimes be partially ineffective. Many patients find dental treatment, even with local analgesia, quite unpleasant. Unlike major surgery, dental treatment is not a rare occurrence, but rather a recurring event in the lives of many. If it is recognized that a very moderate degree of sedation can profoundly influence the situation, virtually wiping out most of the unpleasant limitations of local analgesia, the attitude of the dentist who seeks to give his patients sedation is most laudable. Whatever he does however, he must recognize its dangers and be able to avoid or to deal with them. With this object in view, some of the main ways in which sedation may be given will now be outlined.

ORAL SEDATION

This has been mentioned already as self-administered by the patient, and many patients will doubtless continue to do this, though they should be advised to tell the dentist what they take. As to oral sedation prescribed by the dentist, there is a tendency to suggest that this is unreliable and ineffective. At least some failures however, are directly attributable to neglect of elementary pharmacology. If oral sedation is carefully used, to such effect that the patient, although sedated, can proceed on his own to the dentist and back, and can keep behaving in a socially acceptable way, the procedure will be known as safe and acceptable. Safe, because it will have an extremely low mortality and morbidity, and acceptable because such ill effects as may result will most likely be attributed to another cause—e.g. to a motor vehicle 'accident', the preceding ingestion of a sedative may pass unnoticed. The main problems in prescription of effective sedation by mouth are twofold: firstly to determine the appropriate dose, and then to see that the timing and circumstances of its administration ensure that it has its effect at the right time.

The key to solution of these problems is to take an adequate history, asking about the patient's body weight and general health, and about effects of previously administered drugs. The answers may provide a starting point for appropriate selection of drug and dosage. Anxiety may radically slow the absorption of a drug given orally on the morning of a dental appointment: a dose given on the previous evening may start to allay anxiety and aid sleep. More important this dose can be used as a 'test dose'. Suppose this is a tablet of diazepam 5 mg, that it is taken a while before retiring, and that it produces no obvious objective or subjective effects in the way of ataxia, or slowness of thought or speech. On the following morning the adult patient can safely take two tablets, each diazepam 5 mg, between one and two hours before the time of appointment and arrive well relaxed and in a frame of mind to be agreeable to treatment. This concept of giving three units, one as a test dose and preliminary sedative on the evening before, and one or two to be taken according to the result of the test dose, is good. It has the virtue of pharmacological soundness and achieves safety with maximum chance of an effective dosage being given at first attempt. If satisfactory patient acceptance of treatment can be achieved with oral sedation, its advantages are great: working conditions are excellent because the patient is merely relaxed, and is fully conscious and co-operative. The main danger is the one hinted at earlier, the risk of exposing patients to traffic when their alertness is impaired. This is a risk of any form of sedation which is practised on an out-patient basis, and needs to be assiduously guarded against.

Intra-muscular injection

This has not been a popular route for administration of dental sedation, despite the fact that it can be very satisfactory. It is used to some extent in patients who are hospital in-patients, and will be dealt with under that heading in Chapter 11. It will not be further mentioned at this juncture.

INTRAVENOUS SEDATION

The most that can be done in the way of definition of this procedure is to state that it consists in the injection by the intravenous route, of drugs which depress the state of consciousness, to the end that dental treatment may be facilitated, or at least rendered more acceptable to the patient. There are so many ways in which this has been carried out, and the conscious state of the patient under different methods is so variable, that some description must initially be given of a variety of techniques, in order to convey some idea of what is involved. For this reason a number of techniques will receive mention in this chapter, of which some will be afforded more detailed exposition later.

Credit for the original concept, and for its painstaking development and application over a period of years must go to Professor N. B. Jorgensen of Loma Linda University Dental School in California (Jorgensen *et al* 1963). In outline, his technique involves the slow, careful intravenous injection of drugs, in doses determined by observation of patient response, to induce relaxation, tranquillity and amnesia. Following this, extensive dental treatment whether surgical or restorative may be carried out using adequate local analgesia. The procedure gains ready acceptance by patients, even by those who usually dread dental treatment. The patient is largely amnesic, and so detached from his surroundings as to be partly unaware of the passage of time: a prolonged treatment session may appear to have been quite brief. The 'hangover' from this means of sedation is such that the patient can do little for the rest of the day. In Jorgensen's hands at Loma Linda, this technique with almost no variation, has given highly consistent, good to excellent results over a period of some 25 years. It has not been reported as being widely used elsewhere.

A modern counterpart, in that it is an intravenous drug, which is used more widely by dentists, and with which the patient generally remains conscious and able to respond is intravenous diazepam (Valium-Roche). It is sometimes described as a 'modified Jorgensen technique', although not by that author. Diazepam alone is used, being given by slow intravenous injection until the patient is in a suitably relaxed state, following which local anaesthetic injections are placed, and surgery or restoration proceeds. The dentist works on a tranquil patient who will have little memory of the procedure. Following this technique also, there is a fairly prolonged 'hangover' but with this difference, the patient may appear, within an hour or two of the injection, to have recovered and to be mentally normal, but may, if allowed out on his own, exhibit a quite remarkable irresponsibility of behaviour, and may have a high degree of amnesia as well. A few general comments will be made now on important features of these techniques, but both methods will be considered in depth in Chapter 9.

Diazepam sedation

The introduction of diazepam used in this manner has been responsible, probably more than any other factor, for a tremendous increase in the use of intravenous sedation by dental practitioners working 'single handed'. When one sees diazepam skilfully administered by a careful dentist to a healthy patient, for extensive restorations under local analgesia, one is inclined to feel that it is the answer to the dentist's prayer: the perfect sedative. Dosage appears to be controllable, patients remain easily rousable and able to co-operate, even when at the end of the procedure amnesia is well nigh complete. There are, unfortunately, certain drawbacks inherent in the drug, it is important to recognize precisely to what these are due. The belief is sometimes expressed that research will surely produce a drug which has the advantages of diazepam but is free of its handicaps (Foreman 1972a).

Of the two major problems of diazepam, the more important is its prolonged after effect. To regard this as being an unfortunate failing associated with an otherwise excellent drug is quite mistaken, as a consideration of fundamental pharmacology shows. The basic reason for a single intravenous dose of a drug exerting a fairly steady effect for a period of time, is its slow removal from its field of action, whether this be by distribution, breakdown or excretion. The rate of removal of a drug is proportional to its existing level in body fluids: the graph of the declineof blood level, with passage of time, following a single intravenous dose is an hyperbola. In the case of a drug with a short 'half-life', the early gradient will be steep and the total effect short, but where the half-life is long, the gradient is shallow, the fall in concentration slow, and the effect inevitably prolonged (Fig. 37). Slow removal of the drug is the only pharmacological mechanism which will provide a prolonged, fairly steady state of sedation, and this property also guarantees a prolongation of action beyond the clinically useful stage.

The other adverse feature of diazepam relates to its slow and insidious onset of action on intravenous injection. Despite careful observation, its effects may be minimally obvious even when it is producing quite marked action in the way of amnesia and relaxation. Both of these features render difficult the giving of an accurate appropriate dose for a given patient. Careful observation of the various degrees of ptosis induced by administration of the drug will frequently give some guide to the level of sedation, but this is not invariable, nor is it always easy to interpret.

It is often stated that the safety of intravenous sedation lies largely in the precision of dosage allowed by this route of administration. It is implied or stated that the drug can be 'titrated' against the patient's response, to produce just the degree of sedation required (Foreman 1972b), as if this were a process with all the delightful simplicity and exactitude of adding measured amounts of acid from a burette, to an alkaline solution, and watching for the colour change of an indicator. This is a potentially dangerous over simplification in relation to intravenous administration of any drug, but most of all in relation to those drugs most commonly used for sedation techniques. The difficulties encountered in judging the effects of diazepam have been mentioned. In regard to pentobarbitone (Nembutal-Abbott), the agent used in the Jorgensen technique to determine patient response to sedation, there is a similar problem. This drug had some

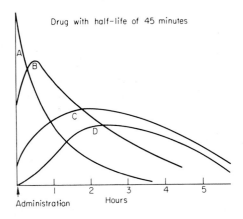

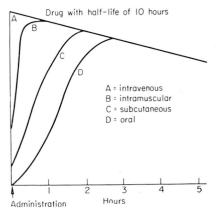

Fig. 37. These graphs illustrate the reasons for fundamental differences in duration of effect of drugs with a short half-life (e.g., methohexitone) and those with a long half-life (e.g., diazepam). The slow onset of effect with oral administration is also shown, as is the need for higher oral doses to obtain a comparable effect. (From Bowman, Rand & West.)

popularity about twenty years ago as a basal sedative agent for patients having diagnostic procedures such as pneumo-encephalography. Its use in this manner has now been largely abandoned, chiefly for the reason that it is extremely difficult to assess, by patient response, the point at which a safe dosage, but one which will provide adequate sedation, has been administered.

METHOHEXITONE IN DENTAL SEDATION

Difficulties such as those outlined have led the protagonists of dental sedation to seek other agents. A drug which is probably more widely used today than most others for this purpose is methohexitone sodium: it will be considered here as epitomizing both the advantages and the problems of a quick-acting, short-acting depressant of consciousness. With this drug there is much greater potential for accurate assessment of the initial dose requirement: its effects are decisive and are seen within little more than 'one circulation time'—generally well within thirty seconds. The short clinical duration of action of modest doses is due to distribution within the body: therefore, provided that the total dosage is kept low, recovery will be quick. The inevitable concomitant disadvantage, the need for constant assessment of the patient's conscious state, and repetitive administration of incremenal doses, to maintain sedation is the main contentious point in the use of short acting agents. Claims for safety are made by the 'operator anaesthetist'—these are greeted with incredulity by the specialist anaesthetist. It is important to examine this use of methohexitone in a little detail if it is to be comprehensible—for the specialist anaesthetist in particular.

The idea of using unsupplemented intravenous anaesthesia for extraction or even restoration of teeth sounds quite incredible to the anaesthetist. He knows that it would be necessary to give dangerously high doses to abolish patient response and this would make maintenance of airway and pulmonary ventilation barely feasible, and the whole procedure most unsafe. The key to the problem, in essence, is that the dentist giving intravenous sedation does not seek to abolish patient response, merely by administration of a central depressant drug. This sort of use of unsupplemented intravenous anaesthesia is not new. Some twenty-five or thirty years ago thiopentone was commonly used as a sole agent to provide general anaesthesia for a wide variety of surgical procedures, including repair of hernia, appendicectomy, reduction of fractures, and many others. The basis of success was that surgeon and anaesthetist worked as a team, a small increment of anaesthetic being injected in anticipation of any stage of the surgical procedure which might be expected to produce a response from the patient. The surgeon had also, of course, to put up with a variable amount of movement by the patient.

The use of intravenous anaesthesia for dentistry has some similarity to this. The dentist, however, starts with some advantage over the conventionally trained surgeon in this regard. The dental surgeon generally has been brought up to work on conscious patients and, at least some of the time, without the aid of local analgesia. He is constantly aware that what he does may cause pain, and may lead to patient response to this pain, his whole outlook and his method and manner of working is constantly geared to this. The anaesthetist is accustomed to catering for the needs of a surgeon who expects to have a quiescent, unresponsive patient on which to operate and who is generally unwilling to take steps to modify surgical stimulation at any point, or indeed frequently incapable of so doing, because of the nature of the surgical procedure.

When a dentist who has had conventional training and experience comes to work with his patient under some form of light sedation, he is better equipped to manage the situation than would be the case if he were accustomed to having no response by the patient to his work. If the dentist proceeds 'with the consideration which would be afforded to a patient having similar work [done] without anaesthesia', (Drummond Jackson 1971a) he will readily achieve much in the way of cavity preparation under very light sedation. Patient acceptance can be expected to be excellent, because of the amnesia and mild euphoria induced by the barbiturate.

It is difficult to emphasize enough the fundamental importance of this concept. The dentist performing restorative work can and does regulate and vary the intensity and timing of painful stimuli to encourage acceptance by the patient. This is the key to success of many forms of ultra-light anaesthesia and sedation in their use for restorative dentistry. A grasp of this fact may enable the anaesthetist to comprehend and give credence to a procedure which has all too often appeared to him to be quite incredible.

Methods of sedation with methohexitone

In this general consideration of the use of methohexitone as a sedative agent, one further point remains to be made. The drug is used in many different ways, and the state of the patient may vary from a fairly constant light sedation to intermittently deep general anaesthesia. No pretence is made that it is possible to elucidate fully this matter, but it is necessary to make a few points, if only to clarify the situation for the benefit of the anaesthetist who is, as a rule, unfamiliar with the use of drugs for sedation procedures, and ignorant of the tremendous potential in such a use of drugs.

An extreme case may serve to illustrate a point. The patient who is recovering consciousness after a brief operation performed under intravenous anaesthesia will be, for a time, in a state which could be described as 'sedation'. The anaesthetist knows, however, that if at this stage a sucker nozzle or something similar be put in the patient's mouth, he will usually react vigorously by turning his head away and by pushing the intruding object away with his hands. Having had experience of this type, the anaesthetist is apt to wonder how such a state of sedation or very light anaesthesia can possibly be of any value in dentistry. The answer to this may be suggested by consideration of a different situation. If a nervous patient is gently made comfortable, reclining in a dental chair, and a small intravenous dose of methohexitone is slowly given, to the accompaniment of soothing reassurance, the patient will generally subside into a relaxed tranquil state in which he will offer no resistance at all to examination and to use of instruments in the mouth. It is this sort of state, induced by a combination of gentle, considerate, understanding handling of the patient, supplemented by intravenous injection of a drug, which constitutes 'intravenous sedation' at its best. A patient in this state, however, will still react in some measure to pain, and the reaction will be by movement, by crying out, or phonation of some sort. The very crux of the problem of intravenous sedation is found in this situation, how best to deal with these reactions to painful stimulation?

Patient response to pain

It may be feasible, if the patient is well sedated, for a skilled and gentle dentist so to regulate and distribute the painful segments of his work, that he can effect cavity preparation without undue patient disturbance, and in such a manner that the patient has a complete amnesia for the procedure. This would be the ideal, its realization is dependent upon a suitable patient, a skilful dentist, and sound patient 'handling'.

Failing this approach, it may be decided that the best line of management is to cease to rely entirely on suggestion and sedation and to administer local analgesia: this also is a very safe and satisfactory solution. Even if a small increment of intravenous methohexitone is also given to maintain sedation, the procedure will still be essentially safe if the patient's state of consciousness is not depressed beyond the stage of ability to respond purposively to the spoken word.

The third alternative is to administer an incremental dose of methohexitone. This is probably the course most commonly adopted. Its results can vary from very satisfactory to highly dubious, and the procedure can be safe or dangerous according to small variations in the manner of administration, the dose given, and the precise indications for the dose. It is these factors, more than any others, which determine the safety or otherwise of this manner of providing sedation for dental treatment. Many considerations indicate plainly that, despite what they may have been taught to do or not to do, a number of dentists using this technique do in fact induce intermittently, in many of their patients, a state of surgical anaesthesia, by their mode and dosage in giving increments of methohexitone. There are three lines of evidence which strongly support this contention.

Dangers of methohexitone sedation

The investigation of the Birmingham group is relevant (Wise *et al* 1969). The electro-encephalographic studies by these workers plainly indicated that the rather high incremental doses which they used were sufficient to induce a state of intermittent general anaesthesia and, not unnaturally, they also demonstrated respiratory depression, depression of protective reflexes, liability to respiratory obstruction and cardiovascular changes which would be expected in fluctuating general anaesthesia induced by methohexitone used as a sole agent for a dental procedure.

The next consideration is that unduly large incremental doses will add up to an unduly large total dose for a given period. The most reliable indication of an unduly large total dose is, unfortunately, retrospective; it is manifest as a marked delay in full recovery of consciousness. In a survey of the use by dentists of the sedation technique known as 'Minimal Increment Methohexitone' involving almost half a million administrations (Drummond Jackson, 1971b) the incidence of various complications, as elicited by answers to a questionnaire, was shown to be extremely low. The complication with the highest recorded incidence—although this was only one in five hundred—was recovery prolonged over one hour. This observation suggests that the aspect of this sedation technique, in which the greatest difficulty arises, is in determination of the correct size and timing of incremental doses. There is no doubt that the skilled, alert, knowledgeable dentist can assess very accurately what is the need, and can give the requisite low dosage, but when it comes to making specific recommendations as to how to judge this, what signs to look for, it is difficult to give sound guidance: this difficulty may be illustrated by reference to movement by a patient in response to a painful stimulus.

If, in response to a slight stimulus, there is a pursing up of the lips and a thrusting by the tongue, this is a fairly good indication that the patient is lightly sedated, and that a further small increment may safely be given. A rather more general, non-purposive movement however, in response particularly to a stronger stimulus, this is a reaction which may be present at even a deep level of general anaesthesia by methohexitone alone. The error of giving repeated increments in an attempt to curb this type of response is probably a major cause of delayed recovery in this procedure, and one of the greatest sources of danger inherent in it. There is also an additional hazard. When a dentist administers an incremental dose, with a view to stopping response to pain, he will be, as it were, poised ready to cut a cavity as soon as the dose takes effect. The patient's descent into anaesthesia with concomitant depression of breathing, risk of respiratory obstruction, and of depression of reflex activity, will occur at the very time when the dentist is concentrating to the full on technical procedures on the teeth. It is at this stage that the dentist cannot, in the true sense, double as operator and anaesthetist: if he is concentrating on his dental work then the watching of the patient will, at this most critical stage, be delegated usually to a nurse. Without passing judgment one merely draws attention to what seems to be an inescapable truth.

A number of features have been mentioned here as being unreliable as indicators for incremental dosage: is there any reliable indicator? There is certainly no simple, straightforward, easily described guide to dosage. In making the assessment of what dose to give and when, a number of factors must be given due consideration. The degree of stimulus which elicits a response must be noted (Drummond Jackson 1971a), also the type of response which is thereby elicited as mentioned above: these will indicate the need for an increment. The size of dose and rate of administration need then to be decided. Here one will have in mind the age, physique, temperament and body weight of the patient, what type of response was seen to an initial dose, and how long did it persist. A running computation has to be mentally kept of dosage so far, of increments given and their effects, with a mental note that to obtain a similar effect to the first, with a second or subsequent increment, dosage will need to be progressively reduced.

As a result of watching a number of dentists acting as operator-anaesthetist one has become convinced that it takes a man of rather exceptional ability to perform really well in this field, to perform these tasks safely, and to obtain consistently good results with safety. When the average dentist attempts to emulate such virtuosity, the result, instead of an even state of sedation, is all too often a series of relatively uncontrolled plunges into deep anaesthesia. The survival of a patient in these circumstances must depend upon his good health and reserve of function: on the capacity to increase cardiac output to compensate for adverse circulatory effects, on the ability of his respiratory drive to overcome minor airway obstruction (Wise *et al,* 1969).

The unphysiological practices which were part of the 'Gas Room' in the past have been noted in Chapters 1 and 3. There was a very low mortality from these procedures, but dental surgery suffered as a result of the poor operating conditions which put a premium on speed, and patients suffered ill effects which were quite unsuspected for long periods.

It will be indeed tragic if misplaced enthusiasm and over-confidence lead to a misuse of intravenous sedation, perhaps comparable with the manner in which the followers of the great McKesson failed to emulate his exceptional skill when using a restricted oxygen supply with nitrous oxide administration (Kaye *et al.* 1946).

CHAPTER 8
NITROUS OXIDE SEDATION

Nitrous oxide is in every day use as a general anaesthetic: in relation to dentistry however, it tends to be associated in the mind of the anaesthetist with an era of general anaesthesia when hypoxic gas mixtures were used. There seems to be some lack of interest among anaesthetists in the use of nitrous oxide as a sedative agent in dentistry and in other fields. This mode of using nitrous oxide is, in fact, so safe and so full of possibilities that it is vitally necessary that anaesthetists should learn to apply it, by a study of its successful use in dentistry.

The method is that nitrous oxide is inhaled in low concentration, diluted with oxygen or with oxygen and air. A common effective concentration would be 25 per cent nitrous oxide, less may be sometimes effective. Generally 50 per cent nitrous oxide is the maximum concentration employed. The patient should remain conscious, as judged by his ability to make reasonable response to the spoken word. It is a curious fact that this technique has become popular in dentistry and obstetrics but has largely failed to 'catch on' in general hospital practice despite an apparently tremendous potential in fields such as safe pain relief for example in myocardial infarction and performance of painful dressings. This contradictory situation is interesting and an attempt will be made to set out the reasons for it.

PROBLEMS FACING THE ANAESTHETIST

One difficulty may be termed conceptual: the medical anaesthetist refers to the 'analgesic' properties of nitrous oxide, with the implication that the drug is effective in relief of pain. In the case of analgesics which are given by injection, morphine for example, one cause of lack of effect is inadequate size of dose: whereas a 5 mg dose may be inadequate, the administration of 10 mg may be effective. This philosophy should not be applied to nitrous oxide inhalation. Increase of the concentration of nitrous oxide will generally lead to lack of co-operation on the part of the patient. As his conscious restraints are released by its actions, he will naturally exhibit the delirium characteristic of both unrelieved pain and second stage anaesthesia. The dental profession has shown generally a much better understanding of this point. Scandinavian authors (e.g., Persson 1951) coined some years ago the term Hypalgesia, and modern American authors refer to 'Relative Analgesia' (Langa 1968a) or to sedation (Jorgensen and Hayden 1972).

Anaesthetists who work in obstetric hospitals increasingly recognize that nitrous oxide and oxygen used during labour is more of a sedative agent, which allays fear—a supplement to analgesics rather than a pain reliever in itself. The anaesthetist who tries to use nitrous oxide for sedation often tends to use an unduly high concentration of the gas. The apparatus which he is accustomed to use is different from that used in dental sedation. The anaesthetist, with awareness of the low potency of nitrous oxide as an anaesthetic agent, tends to use a full face mask, a flow rate approximating to the patient's minute volume, and a circuit which is free of leaks.

The dentist uses a nasal inhaler with delivery tubes which are often barely adequate to cope with peak inspiratory flow rates (Fig. 38) and to have, on the nasal mask, a device which can admit air to the circuit (Fig. 39). Even in the absence of this deliberate air leak, the use of a nasal mask, along with conditions which do not prohibit mouth breathing, will allow air dilution of the inhaled gas mixture. The important consideration is the inescapable fact that the common cause of lack of success in the use of nitrous oxide as a sedation agent is a lack of appreciation of the nature of the procedure leading, by one means or another, to the administration of an undesirably high concentration of nitrous oxide, with the chief end result of loss of co-operation by the patient. The anaesthetist is, of course, accustomed to dealing with this phenomenon, but because he sees lack of co-operation principally as an incident on the way to achievement of general anaesthesia, he will have a natural tendency to deal with it by deepening the level of unconsciousness. In the use of nitrous oxide as a sedative agent, the only correct procedure at the first sign of lack of co-operation, is to take steps to lighten the plane of sedation, whether by admission of more air or oxygen or by diminution of the flow of nitrous oxide.

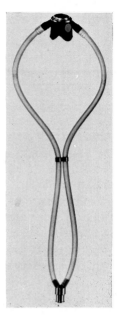

Fig. 38. A nasal inhaler of the type used for dental sedation. The long narrow tubes pass round each side of the patient's head and are the means of retaining the nose-piece as well as of gas delivery. The Y piece incorporates a non-return valve which prevents rebreathing.

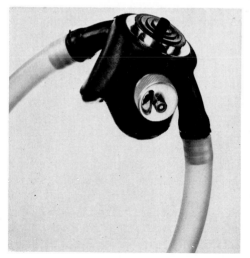

Fig. 39. Close up view of a nose-piece to which is fitted an air intake valve, which may be opened or closed by turning the milled exterior casing.

Apart from the concentration of the gas in the inspired mixture, the most significant feature determining the uptake of nitrous oxide is the patient's effective minute volume of respiration. Any painful or unpleasant stimulus may tend to increase the rate and depth of breathing. In the circuit used by the anaesthetist this automatically and inevitably increases nitrous oxide uptake, usually with onset of delirium, or at least of diminished co-operation. In the case of the eqiupment used for dental sedation, however, because of the narrow-ness of the delivery tubes to the nose-piece and the presence in the nose-piece of the air dilution valve or hole, any tendency for increased depth of sedation to result from a spell of hyperventilation is automatically corrected.

Most of the considerations dealt with in Chapter 7 applying to the performance of dentistry under intravenous sedation apply with equal force to the use of nitrous oxide as a sedative agent. The desirability of using effective local analgesia, the importance of gentleness and care in working—all those factors comprehended in the term 'good patient handling', to which the central sedative effect is no more than a supplement. There is, however, one important difference between the two methods. Whereas some effect can be achieved in diminishing patient response—albeit dangerously—by increasing the depth of intravenous sedation, the attempt to increase the depth of nitrous oxide sedation is generally of no value at all in obtaining patient acceptance of painful treatment. While this may be regarded in some measure as a limitation upon nitrous oxide seda-tion, it certainly constitutes a most important safety factor. This feature, added to the extremely evanescent action of nitrous oxide, which is such that recovery after prolonged inhalation is complete within five minutes or so, make it an ideal agent for fairly routine use for sedation in out-patient dentistry.

LEVELS OF SEDATION

The level of depression of consciousness of patients undergoing nitrous oxide sedation should always be such that the patient is in Stage I according to the classification of Guedel. In this stage con-sciousness is blurred, but not lost, there are no characteristic cardio-vascular changes apart from slight cutaneous vasodilation which may contribute to the comfortable sense of warmth and relaxation described by most patients. The level of sedation is gauged by the patient's responses. He must retain his response to the spoken word, and reaction to pain should be such as indicates that awareness is maintained. Any suggestion of delirium should be taken as an indication to lighten the plane of sedation.

Respiration must be observed routinely, as a reassurance that all is well with the patient as well as to guard against inadvertent deepening of sedation by over-breathing. Rhythmic movement of the reservoir bag should be noted frequently to confirm the integrity of the patient's connection to the apparatus, as well as the continuance of respiration, and adequacy of gas flows. Although deepening of the level of sedation will generally be shown plainly by some failure of co-operation on the part of the patient, e.g., failure to keep the mouth open for treatment (Langa, 1968b), it should not be tacitly assumed that this will always be so. It is quite possible that a patient who slips into a stage of general anaesthesia, will remain quiescent and will keep breathing satisfactorily. Frequently no harm will result from this, but the danger exists that maintenance of a stage of general anaesthesia for a length of time may be followed by vomiting. Such vomiting may be sudden and unheralded, or may follow some stimulus. If the patient is still anaesthetized, vomiting could constitute a hazard, from aspiration of vomited material into the air passages, or from laryngospasm due to glottic irritation by foreign material. It should be stressed again that only conscious response by the patient to the spoken word is a guarantee of a sufficiently light plane of sedation. The administration of a particular concentration of nitrous oxide does not provide any assurance that a patient will remain conscious. In a number of experiments in which healthy male volunteers have undertaken performance of tests under nitrous oxide inhalation (Steinberg and Summerfield 1957) the concentration of nitrous oxide inhaled was 30 per cent: certain volunteers could not participate because inhalation of this low concentration of gas resulted in loss of consciousness.

The desirability of employing local analgesia in conjunction with sedation for all dental work which might cause significant pain, has been mentioned already: it is important that the local analgesia be fully effective. A state of light sedation, while abolishing patient response to stimuli evoking fear or discomfort, will not abolish reaction to pain resulting from inadequacies of local analgesia, rather will it tend to exaggerate any response to infliction of pain. This response is a feature which may be of diagnostic assistance when exploration is undertaken, in a nervous patient, to determine for example, the vitality of the pulp of a suspect tooth. In the patient who is comfortably sedated, the mere procedure of cutting into a tooth is not likely to evoke a misleading, spurious reaction suggesting pain. It is appropriate to emphasize again the fact that patient handling and effective local analgesia are the important features ensuring the success of any sedation technique, without these the central sedation induced by any method will be largely ineffective in facilitating treatment.

A word of explanation is necessary here, for it is about this stage that the casual onlooker at dental sedation may express serious doubts about the whole procedure. These will not now be the initial misgivings about safety, but rather an expression of disbelief about the reality or validity of the concept of sedation. Specialist anaesthetists tend to dismiss nitrous oxide sedation for dentistry as a 'gimmick', senior members of the dental profession may refer to it as a 'crutch' which is needed by some of their colleagues who lack competence in patient management or use of local analgesia. This criticism is unfair and deserves comment. A senior dentist who practises in an urban community may be unaware of the degree to which unintentional selection of patients is exercised in his practice. Capable general practice dentists are frequently in short supply relative to the numbers of well-motivated patients who seek private dental care. If a patient finds the methods of a dentist unacceptable, he will most likely go elsewhere. The dentist is unlikely to notice such a withdrawal as his practice will remain busy. It is easy to be critical of the dentist who employs nitrous oxide sedation in a solo private practice. He may become convinced, and quite correctly so, that the use of sedation makes dental treatment acceptable to difficult patients, and indeed even to those who, without it, are impossible to manage. Because of his circumstances, he has little defence against sceptical colleagues who snipe at him with suggestions which may imply his patients like the sensation of getting 'high' on gas.

The writer has become convinced of the efficacy of sedation: this conviction stems from experience with patients who have been referred for general anaesthesia on account of non-acceptance of treatment with local analgesia. It has been in the case of certain children in particular, where one felt that intravenous induction would be unacceptable and the history suggested that the appearance of the out-patient theatre would frighten the patient, that they have been referred for sedation with nitrous oxide. The regularity with which these difficult patients relax into a tranquil state and accept extensive local analgesic injections needs to be seen to be believed. The procedure is quite evidently safer than full general anaesthesia and therefore must command the attention of the specialty of anaesthesia.

Apparatus used for sedation

Up to this point little mention has been made of the detail of apparatus except to draw certain distinctions between apparatus used by the dentist and that used by the anaesthetist, by way of explanation of some of the difficulties which anaesthetists have met with in attempting this procedure. It is necessary to consider the apparatus in detail, with particular emphasis on means whereby safety is assured when the dentist is performing the surgery as well as managing the sedation.

In former times this type of sedation, or 'analgesia' as it would then have been termed, was effected by attaching to the patient the nose-piece of an intermittent flow, or 'demand flow' type anaesthetic apparatus. This apparatus exhibited one notable feature not found in modern machines, namely, as the patient inhaled, thus triggering the machine to deliver a gas mixture, the machine emitted a very characteristic sound. By this means the expert dentist had an audible indication of the performance of the machine and the state of the patient's respiration. However the disadvantages and limitations of this apparatus have led to its general replacement with apparatus of the continuous flow type. The breathing circuit of this modern apparatus resembles the Magill circuit described in Chapter 3 (Fig. 10, p. 34). Dosage of nitrous oxide is regulated primarily by setting its concentration in the gas mixture which the patient inhales: for example a flow of two litres per minute of nitrous oxide with eight litres per minute of oxygen, will result in a total flow of ten litres per minute and a concentration of twenty per cent nitrous oxide in the inhaled mixture. The other major factor determining uptake of nitrous oxide is the patient's tidal ventilation. The dentist must be constantly aware, in the background as it were, of the patient's tidal volume and rate of respiration, to detect marked changes which can lead to significant variations in level of sedation.

TECHNIQUE OF NITROUS OXIDE SEDATION

A flow of oxygen approximating to the patient's estimated minute volume (some ten litres per minute in an adult) is started and the nose-piece gently applied: the exhale valve should be free and the air intake valve on the nose-piece should be closed at this stage. For some two minutes or more, at least on his first visit, the patient should be allowed to breathe pure oxygen. This will serve to let him become accustomed to the apparatus, but more important, it will show up any faults harmlessly, and will also reveal the occasional patient who may be adversely affected by this technique of sedation: this point will be enlarged upon later. A normal patient should be able to breathe oxygen without any obvious effect. Any upset which is not immediately remedied by gentle reassurance, perhaps with momentary removal of the nose-piece, should be a warning to desist until the explanation of the upset is determined and the situation remedied. All being well, at this stage the flow of nitrous oxide is commenced to give a concentration at first of some ten per cent. The concentration is then gradually increased, over a period of two minutes or more, to a level at which the patient exhibits or experiences a slight but definite effect from the gas. The desirable effects are a sensation of warmth, comfort and relaxation, perhaps with some sensation of numbness or tingling in the extremities and about the mouth and face. The patient's consciousness will be slightly obtunded and his responses a little slow. The concentration of nitrous oxide in the inhaled mixture at which these effects occur should be noted carefully as providing a general indication of the degree of response of this particular patient to nitrous oxide, which even if not constant, at least follows a fairly consistent pattern. Nitrous oxide sedation is, of course, ideal for use in repetitive treatments: it is worthwhile noting carefully all details of the response of an individual patient, their preference for slow or rapid introduction of the gas, for example. On the first occasion introduction of nitrous oxide should always be slow. On future occasions, an experienced dentist may, for a suitable patient, safely effect a quicker induction of sedation if this is in keeping with the desires of the patient.

Use of special apparatus

Sedation with nitrious oxide can be effected readily by using a standard continuous flow anaesthetic apparatus to which is attached a dental type nose-piece. However, if the dentist is to carry out sedation simultaneously with performance of dental surgery, it is essential that certain safety features be incorporated into the apparatus to effect two specific safeguards. The first prevents the delivery of a mixture containing less than a predetermined level of oxygen, be it 25 per cent, 30 per cent or 50 per cent. The second guards against failure or relative inadequacy of rate of supply of gas mixture to the patient. It ensures that if this occurs, the patient will automatically and freely inhale air.

Some of the safety features which are now so highly developed in dental sedation apparatus should find acceptance with medical anaesthetists. This is an area in which dental anaesthesia has valuable safety lessons to teach to the discipline of anaesthesia. The simplest form of oxygen supply safety device is exemplified in the 'McKesson Analor' and the 'Quantiflex R.A.' (Fig. 40) machines. Each of these has an 'ON-OFF' switch: when the flow of gases is started by this switch, with the fine adjustment valves for each gas closed, there is immediate delivery of oxygen at $2\frac{1}{2}$ litres per minute. The flow can be increased above this, but cannot be reduced below $2\frac{1}{2}$ litres per minute except by turning off all gas delivery.

Further, the flow of nitrous oxide is dependent upon availability of oxygen: if the oxygen flow fails, from any cause, nitrous oxide delivery is automatically and simultaneously discontinued. As the maximum flow of nitrous oxide approximates to eight litres per minute, this device safeguards against the possible administration of an hypoxic mixture.

In dental sedation apparatus, provision is made to ensure that re-breathing, in and out of the reservoir bag, cannot occur. When the standard Magill circuit is used for general anaesthesia re-breathing is prevented, or its degree regulated, by adjustment of the gas delivery flow rate relative to the minute volume of the patient. Because re-breathing in dental sedation is neither necessary nor desirable, it is usually prevented by the incorporation in the circuit of a non-return valve, allowing of inhalation from the reservoir bag but preventing exhalation into it: the entire expired gas from the patient must go out via the exhale valve on the nose-piece. The non-return valve is often

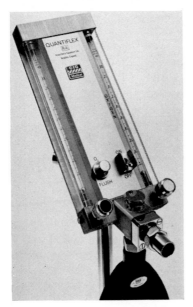

Fig. 40. The Quantiflex R.A. machine uses as a safety measure against hypoxia a constant $2\frac{1}{2}$ litres per minute of oxygen which flows as soon as any gas is turned on by the switch shown at lower right.

incorporated in the bag mount of the apparatus—where it is a permanent fixture and is not readily removed. An alternative used in apparatus made by Commonwealth Industrial Gases (Australia) is to place the valve in the 'Y' junction, to the limbs of which attach the delivery tubes of the nasal mask. When the nose-piece is removed, and replaced by a standard full face mask with exhale valve, the circuit reverts to the standard Magill circuit, and can be effectively employed for general anaesthesia or resuscitation.

Safeguard against failure or inadequacy of the gas supply from any cause is provided by an air intake valve on the gas supply side of the reservoir bag. If the patient's inhalation is sufficient to empty the reservoir bag, whether the reason be increased ventilation by the patient or diminution of the gas flow, this valve allows the patient to inhale freely atmospheric air. A useful refinement is to have a simple 'whistle' incorporated in this air intake so that the dentist receives an unmistakable audible warning as soon as there is entrainment of air from relative inadequacy of gas flow (Fig. 41).

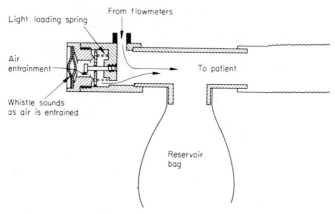

Fig. 41.   Sectional diagram of the head of the 'Entonox' apparatus made by Commonwealth Industrial Gases, Australia, to show the air entrainment valve with whistle. In this apparatus the non-return valve is not a fixture—it is situated in the Y piece of the nasal inhaler.

Safety of the procedure

The means of preventing administration of an hypoxic gas mixture has been mentioned: it is of such fundamental importance that it will now be dealt with in more detail. In addition to the apparatus already described in this connection there is a more sophisticated one in which, although nitrous oxide and oxygen are delivered through separate flow meters, the controls are not the usual two fine adjustment valves. There is one control for total flow, and a separate milled wheel which is moved to vary the oxygen percentage, by simultaneous alteration in the flow rate of nitrous oxide and oxygen. The Quantiflex M.D.M. is such an apparatus (Fig. 42), it is made in two models— one with a lower limit of 50 per cent oxygen, for dental sedation, and one which goes as low as 30 per cent oxygen for general anaesthesia. It is simple in appearance, but it is a sophisticated piece of equipment, any interruption to oxygen flow immediately cuts off the nitrous oxide. It might be expected that it would need frequent servicing, but one which has been in use for some time in a busy outpatient theatre has proved to be robust and reliable.

As an alternative to ensuring an adequate oxygen supply by use of special flow meters, one can use simple flow meters, and instead of having nitrous oxide supplied pure in a cylinder, use a cylinder which

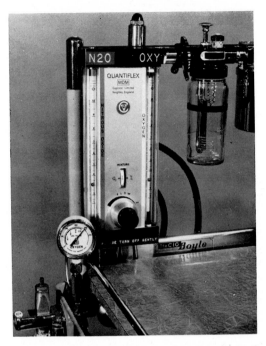

Fig. 42. The Quantiflex M.D.M. flowmeter, fitted to the Boyle machine in the out-patient theatre, Royal Dental Hospital of Melbourne. It is used routinely for general anaesthesia.

contains nitrous oxide already mixed, in equal proportion by volume, with oxygen. The protection against hypoxia is here supplied by pre-mixing the oxygen with the gas. When this mixture is delivered from the apparatus and mixed with oxygen from a separate supply, any concentration of nitrous oxide from 0 to 50 per cent can be attained, but never more than 50 per cent nitrous oxide. There is complete freedom from any anxiety that failure of apparatus will allow of delivery of an hypoxic mixture. The only limitation on reliability of this premixed gas and oxygen, now marketed for several years under the name of 'Entonox', is a predictable one. In a cylinder of Entonox exposed to extreme low temperatures of minus 6° to minus 8° Celsius, 'layering' of nitrous oxide occurs. If the cylinder is used without first allowing it to re-warm, and then mixing the contents by agitation, there may be delivery initially of an oxygen rich mixture, and later of one with less than 50 per cent oxygen in it. With this one reservation,

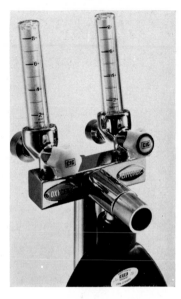

Fig. 43. Apparatus for administration of Entonox for Dental Sedation:
its simplicity is evident. A sectional diagram of the head as shown in
Figure 41.

use of Entonox gives high reliability and safety with the simplest of
apparatus (Fig. 43).

Selection of apparatus

When a dentist decides to employ this form of sedation in his practice
he is faced with the need to make a choice from various types of
apparatus for administration of nitrous oxide. This is a decision which
is as full of problems as purchase of a motor car, in either case an
awareness of pitfalls is of assistance. A fundamental point is that the
performance of a gas apparatus should be judged in the context of its
use by the dentist on patients and not chiefly by its performance in
any other circumstances.

If a dentist is associated with a school where sedation is established
and practised on a sound basis, he will have ample opportunity for
such an assessment. If, however, he does not have such access, he may
be subject to undesirable pressures of salesmanship.

There is sometimes formed an association between study groups or societies within the profession, who seek to advance knowledge of sedation, and distributors of equipment. This is natural and acceptable—if the dentist finds certain equipment to his liking he is justified in recommending it to his colleagues. It is common for conventions to be held by professional societies or groups to introduce dentists to sedation. These may include lectures and demonstrations but an important feature in most is that dentists new to sedation are encouraged to experience the effect of nitrous oxide on themselves. This is a practice which is said by most teachers to be desirable, and as part of the education of the dentist has something to commend it: it should not go beyond mere appreciation of the subjective sensations associated with low concentrations of nitrous oxide.

These experiments are sometimes taken much further than this, however. One is aware of cases in which dentists have been given increasing concentrations of nitrous oxide over a short period of time, and their response tested to a sharp probe on the gingival margin. Quite predictably, a concentration of nitrous oxide well in excess of 50 per cent may be needed to achieve obtunding of such sensation within a short time (five minutes or less). It is necessary to make quite clearly the point that this type of quick induction of analgesia or general anaesthesia is not the objective in safe administration of nitrous oxide sedation. The figures obtained from results of such an 'experiment' have sometimes been exhibited to suggest the desirability of purchase of a sedation apparatus capable of delivering nitrous oxide in a concentration exceeding 50 per cent: this is felt to be not a sound basis on which to promote the sale of any particular type of sedation apparatus.

Condition of the patient

Safety factors considered to this point have been concerned with guarding against technical mishap. It is now necessary to consider whether there are medical considerations which would militate against safety or success of nitrous oxide sedation in any patients. It is a drug which is almost unique in its lack of undesirable toxic effects: up to date the only one which has been definitely noted is that which may result from continued administration for twenty-four hours or more, namely depression of bone marrow function leading to blood dyscrasia. Even in repetitive administrations there have been no toxic effects demonstrated, although they are being sought diligently because of increasing recognition of the occurrence of toxic effects on repeated administration at short intervals of various volatile anaesthetic agents. In spite of intensive investigation, nitrous oxide has so far retained its remarkable reputation of being almost non-toxic.

This is not, of course, to say that sedation with this agent will invariably be successful. Two of the commonest causes of failure are fairly directly related to its psychotropic effects. The patient who is accustomed to taking alcohol in quantity and to enjoying its effects may not be amenable to satisfactory sedation by this agent. It is not that he will find the experience unpleasant, but it is unlikely that much dentistry will be achieved. There is another class of patient for whom nitrous oxide is unsuitable—this is a patient who finds the sensations associated with induction of sedation unpleasant. Sometimes this is a relatively minor subjective complaint, and an experienced dentist can by various means—by slow induction, by reassurance, by demonstration to the patient that the level of sedation is easily controlled, persuade the patient to accept it and induce successful sedation. It is essential to recognize, however, the existence of a small number of patients for whom, it seems, the inhalation of nitrous oxide induces most unpleasant hallucinatory effects (Bergström and Bernstein 1968). Such patients, after induction of anaesthesia or sedation, may be plagued for considerable periods by recurring nightmares; a condition approaching psychosis may result. Dentists who employ nitrous oxide should be aware of the existence of this hazard so that, if it is suspected, the patient can be gently questioned about possible unpleasant effects and, if necessary, the use of the agent discontinued. The use, in its place, of an intravenous agent which quickly produces unconsciousness or at least amnesia, methohexitone for example, may be satisfactory.

Use in the 'poor risk' patient

Apart from these effects however, what of the use of nitrous oxide in this manner in 'poor risk' medical patients? There have been very few reports of problems, but this is not to say that they do not occur. One has had personal or indirect contact with a sufficient number of problems to be keenly aware of the potential for trouble of this technique—it is on this experience that the following observations are

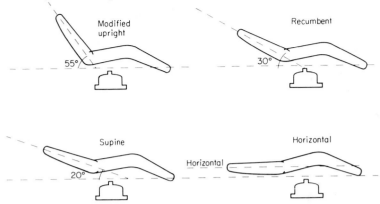

Fig. 44. This shows what is understood by terms which describe various positions of the dentist's contour chair. Only the Horizontal (or even head down) position is acceptable for any procedure which involves depression of consciousness (see also page 162).

chiefly based. In many texts the tenor of remarks is that the high oxygen content of the inspired mixture and retention of consciousness makes the procedure completely safe.

Retention of consciousness is difficult to ensure, however. It is not sufficient merely to keep constant the concentration of gas delivered, for unnoticed hyperventilation from any cause can sharply increase the uptake of nitrous oxide. A number of features have been described as indicating deepening sedation—failure to keep the mouth open, snoring, restlessness or other early signs of delirium—but these are not reliable. A patient may become unconscious without manifesting any of these signs, but remaining quiescent and maintaining apparently normal respiration. The occurrence of overbreathing which deepens the plane of unconsciousness will probably be followed by shallow breathing or even apnoea, and may possibly lead to other events, as suggested by the case history which follows.

A middle-aged male attended for conservative dental treatment with nitrous oxide sedation given as 'Entonox'. His answers to preliminary questions revealed that he was under treatment with Aldomet (methyl-dopa) but suggested that he was in good general health. Nitrous oxide close to fifty per cent with oxygen was given by nasal mask with the air intake valve closed. Shortly after treatment was started it was noticed that the patient was breathing deeply, it was then observed that he was not responding. He was given oxygen to breathe but remained unresponsive for some minutes, then slowly recovered consciousness. For about half an hour he was disorientated and confused and complained of headache. After arrival at his home he was seen by his own doctor who reported to the dentist that his blood pressure was considerably higher than usual.

This case report, although sketchy, gives food for thought. The manner in which the report was made is of interest. The dentist telephoned to enquire if one knew of this apparent incompatability of 'Aldomet' and 'Entonox': his appreciation of the possible causation of mishaps with sedation apparently did not go beyond this concept. The dentist who uses sedation commonly lacks the anaesthetist's awareness and understanding of respiratory physiology and would generally take little notice of fluctuations in tidal volume and rate of respiration. He would be unaware of likely variations in carbon dioxide levels in the blood induced by depression of consciousness with apnoea, which may follow overbreathing. Recent studies in autoregulation of cerebral blood flow summarized in an Editorial (*Lancet* 1973) suggest the need for a change in ideas on hypertensive encephalopathy and describe a mechanism whereby it may be readily induced in the hypertensive patient by hypercapnia. As this patient was not supine, a temporary cerebral anaemia may be invoked as a cause of his symptoms (Bourne, 1957) but perhaps one should not be unduly facile in jumping to this conclusion.

The greatest cause for concern is the question: how many minor episodes of this type, or others, occur and go unreported? The psychology of reporting is significant: any professional man is likely to notice and report conditions which he feels that he understands, and with which he is equipped to deal, but is likely to ignore those which he does not understand. The dentist in this case believed that he was dealing with a simple drug interaction—as such it was comprehensible and he sought further enlightenment.

The average dentist who uses sedation at present will generally have no one to whom he may turn in seeking elucidation of problems and will therefore tend not to report them. If anaesthetists will recognize not only the importance of these methods, but their tremendous potential, and learn to apply them and understand them, the dentist may then have someone to whom to appeal when troubles occur. As a result there may be some chance of studying effectively and of elucidating some of the problems arising in the course of nitrous oxide sedation, rare though they may be.

One has has sufficient experience of sudden unheralded vomiting in patients undergoing sedation for purposes other than dental, to regard it as a real hazard. The occurrence of vomiting in a patient with cardiac decompensation could readily be the start of a potentially lethal hypoxia from respiratory obstruction due to spasm of the glottis. It would be desirable for the dentist to be able to consult with an anaesthetist before embarking on nitrous oxide sedation in poor-risk cardiac patients.

The patient with advanced pulmonary emphysema would be a most unsuitable candidate for this sedation procedure. If he is in a sufficiently advanced state of respiratory failure he may, when given oxygen to breathe, suffer respiratory depression followed by narcosis from elevation of his carbon dioxide level. It will be immediately protested that no-one could fail to recognize a patient in this state of respiratory failure, but experience with patients referred by dentists for general anaesthesia indicates that this can occur. Not every patient with advanced emphysema is big, blue and barrel-chested. The small pale man who suffers from emphysema and who moves about quietly, with a studied economy of effort, may give a laconic answer in the negative if asked about shortness of breath. If given oxygen to breathe, he may quickly exhibit confusion or disorientation. This is one significant reason for emphasis placed upon the importance of giving the patient oxygen to breathe before introducing nitrous oxide. The immediate treatment on occurrence of this complication is to discontinue the oxygen. If any respiratory trouble or depression of consciousness persists, one should attempt gentle intermittent positive pressure ventilation with air, from a recoil bag resuscitator such as the Ambu or the Air Viva.

There is little doubt that nitrous oxide sedation stands out as being the only method which is suitable for repetitive use on a truly ambulatory basis for dental sedation. Nitrous oxide with oxygen is undoubtedly the safest of all available agents for routine use as a sedative agent by dentists in their practice. It is a matter of vital importance, therefore, that such problems as arise with its use, be they major or minor, should be examined minutely and fully elucidated, so that a true perspective may be obtained of the potential of this remarkable technique.

CHAPTER 9
INTRAVENOUS SEDATION

In examining intravenous sedation to seek the means of its safe clinical application it is instructive to consider further the original technique of Jorgensen as applied in the Loma Linda University Dental School Clinic, to see where emphasis is chiefly placed, and to see what is the basis of the excellent record of safety and efficacy of the procedure at that clinic.

The method described and used by Jorgensen is fairly familiar in detail (Jorgensen and Hayden 1972), the important features are outlined: drugs are given by slow intravenous injection, firstly pentobarbitone ('Nembutal'—Abbott), as a solution of 100 mg in 2 ml administered by slow injection of incremental doses, with long pauses between, with the object of being able to observe the earliest effect of the drug on the patient's cerebral function. The dose which produces this first effect is noted, and is used as a guide to further administration of pentobarbitone, and then of pethidine to a maximum of 25 mg and hyoscine to a maximum of 0·32 mg. It is emphasised that during and after the administration of this sedation, the patient should remain conscious. If consciousness be lost, this is an indication for stopping all further procedures whether they be injection of local anaesthetic or performance of surgery, and watching the patient's respiration and circulation until consciousness is regained, before proceeding further.

The intravenous injection of sedative drugs is a part only of intravenous sedation. In the patient who has an unreasoning fear or emotion, mere injection of these or other drugs may produce a blurring of consciousness which causes restlessness and loss of co-operation. Unless the cause of such reaction is recognized, the dentist may be misled into administration of further drug in an endeavour to control restlessness, and may thus induce general anaesthesia, with its attendant risks from loss of protective responses. The student of the Loma Linda clinic would be unlikely to make such an error. By precept and example he gains a high degree of expertise in gentle and considerate patient handling to which sedation by drugs is no more than a supplement.

When the patient has been settled by quiet suggestion and by careful sedation and is in a satisfactory condition, local analgesia is induced to cover the entire procedure intended. It is important to note that very much more stress in both practice and in graduate and undergraduate teaching, is placed by Professor Jorgensen upon meticulous perfection in local analgesic technique than is placed upon the intravenous sedation itself. He treats local analgesia as an important clinical discipline based on anatomy, physiology and pharmacology. He has anatomical specimens of skulls, maxillae, and mandibles and carefully preserved dissections to illustrate normal anatomy and variations relating to every type of local injection used in dentistry. He insists upon the use of needles which are sufficiently stout and robust to be used to palpate bony landmarks, with a view to ensuring perfection of anatomical placement of solution. In order that these rather large needles may be painlessly introduced there is insistence on adequate topical analgesic being applied, after drying the mucous membrane, and some time before injection. There is emphasis on the importance of making an immediate small injection of solution after introduction of the needle and on its very slow advancement, preceded by small depositions of the solution.

In this clinic which is so widely renowned for its intravenous sedation, there is, in general, less clinical emphasis on the sedation than upon local analgesia. Intravenous injection is made by the student in routine fashion under close supervision, while an experienced nurse sees to airway care by posture of the head and support of the jaw.

Anaesthetists who have read of Jorgensen's routine use by intravenous injection of pentobarbitone, pethidine and hyoscine have generally expressed surprise that these potent agents could be used by dentists routinely for safe achievement of sedation. The answer lies in the manner of their use. The clinic staff show a wonderful dedication to the needs of the patient, and dosage of sedative drugs can be minimal, with good effect. The procedure is supervised closely by Professor Jorgensen and others who are experienced practical anaesthetists. Teaching is directed to avoiding trouble, their almost intuitive knowledge of patients assists this, and the capability is always present of dealing with airway and other problems should they arise.

The environment is such that the procedure is extremely safe, but this does not necessarily mean that the safety resides either in the choice of drugs or in the rules by which they are administered.

DIAZEPAM

The use of diazepam given by intravenous injection as a prelude to a session of dental treatment under local analgesia, constitutes a technique which is similar in many aspects to the Loma Linda technique, but which is, because of the unique pharmacology of the drug, very much safer. The pharmacology of diazepam is the chief factor contributing to this safety, in particular the wide margin, in healthy patients, between the effective dose and the one which causes a dangerous depression of vital functions. Its major disadvantage has been noted already, its prolonged after effect or hangover—an inevitable concomitant of its most desirable virtue, that a single intravenous injection is followed by one hour or more of satisfactory sedation.

It was observed early in this section that no sedation technique could be truly labelled 'safe'—the ideal is that any type of dental sedation procedure should be carried out only by a person who has adequate training to recognize and to deal effectively with any possible complications. Conditions inevitably fall short of this ideal, and dentists with sound motivation but with barely adequate training will use intravenous sedation, therefore the basic safety of diazepam and of other methods needs to be critically examined. This will be done in three sections.

The general health of the patient

In assessment of the medical status of the patient the dental practitioner is at a disadvantage, and likely to remain so. The dentist is not a physician, and does not practise medicine. No matter what has been his training or education in the sphere, the taking of a history of clinical symptoms which may suggest general disease, the making of a general physical examination, and the integration of these to formulate a diagnosis is not what the dentist is accustomed to doing. Nor is it sufficient for a dental practitioner merely to ask a list of questions about symptoms as does the physician. It would be analogous to a doctor taking a mouth mirror and probe and examining a mouth as would a dentist—he could not be relied upon to give a sound assessment of any dental condition, other than gross caries.

The best practice for the dentist to follow is to ask questions about his patient's current and past medical treatment and illnesses along factual lines, questions such as those set out in the Questionnaire shown in Fig. 27, Chapter 6. A series of negative answers to questions of this sort is strongly suggestive of good health. If this is followed up by a conversational series of questions about the patient's daily activity, the answers to which indicate a capability to walk up hills and upstairs without dyspnoea, the likelihood is very strong that the patient is sufficiently healthy to undergo sedation and dental treatment safely.

Any preanaesthetic medical assessment of a patient, however thorough, is essentially provisional in nature. In the hands of the careful anaesthetist the intial stages of any anaesthetic administration are conducted with the mental reservation that, if an atypical or adverse reaction is shown to any drug administration, he will desist, at least temporarily. Thus it is that the assessment of the patient's health overlaps with the next stage.

Reaction of the patient to drug administration

Intravenous administration of drugs has a two-edged nature. If the administration is carefully carried out using appropriately sized and slowly given increments, there is a high degree of safety inherent in the technique. The potential exists, however, for a quicker, more effective administration of a dangerously large dose than is possible by almost any other means. At the hands of the dentist, the medical assessment of the patient may be less than complete. It is, therefore, doubly important that the administration of the drug, to test the response of the patient, be carried out with scrupulous care. The dentist needs to be meticulous in the initial administration of a suitably small test dose, and to wait an adequate period to see its effect, and should know what to look for. In the case of diazepam, a suitable test dose for an adult would be 2·0 mg: that is less than one half millilitre of the usual solution of 'Valium' (Roche). This should be injected slowly, and it is necessary to be clear as to the reason for this. The objective is to avoid a rapid increase in the concentration of the drug in the blood. A small dose injected quickly can produce such an effect, in that a certain portion of the blood proceeding through heart and lungs to the brain will have in it an unduly high concentration of the drug and will produce an effect which is disproportionate to the dose given. The time that it takes for the blood to travel from a vein in the arm to an artery in the brain—the 'arm-brain' circulation time—is a significant interval to have in mind in these circumstances, it is some 18 to 25 seconds normally. If the first 2·0 mg be injected evenly over a space of ten seconds, it will be reaching the brain over the next twenty seconds, its effects may first be seen at about a minute from starting the injection. It is important to look for any sign significant of drug action, and not to rely on any one or two signs or symptoms. It is of little use to ask the patient about subjective sensations of sleepiness—the patient will generally admit only to a slight sense of relaxation. Ptosis—drooping of the eyelids—is a variable sign and not always easy to assess. It is desirable to estimate the patient's whole mental function—this is best done by quietly conversing with the patient about trivia before the injection is commenced, and as it is made. It is important to note any definite change in the patient's manner of speech or expression, whether it be silence or undue talking, it is change which is significant. When this is noted it is an indication to refrain from further dosage until the full effect is seen of what has already been given, then to administer in stages a further dose which is less than half what has already been given, and wait to see its effect.

These instructions represent an attempt to convey something of the rather subtle changes which must be looked for after administration of an intravenous sedation agent, if serious trouble due to overdosage is to be consistently avoided, and a maximum effect obtained safely with the smallest feasible dose. If a method such as that outlined be scrupulously followed, then the patient with significant medical disability—significant in that it increases his sensitivity to the effects of the drug in use—will certainly be recognized before he comes to any harm: and this is surely the prime objective in this exercise. There remains only one further factor to consider.

The state of the patient's vital functions

When the patient is considered to be in a satisfactory state of sedation, it is necessary to check on respiration, circulation and protective reflexes. If in the supine patient, air can be readily detected going in and out of the mouth or nose, then respiration may be considered adequate. The patient should be given a quiet command to 'swallow', obedience to this suggests that protective reflexes are intact. If the colour is pink and circulatory return brisk, all is satisfactory and dental treatment may begin. If there were no response to a request to swallow, the patient would be gently disturbed to wake him up: if this succeeds all is well. It is highly desirable, as stressed by Jorgensen, to ensure that the patient is capable of conscious response before starting to place local analgesic injections and to operate in the mouth.

The injection of local analgesic is a critical phase of the whole procedure, and if it is not carried out using a meticulous technique, and with the utmost care to avoid infliction of pain, the success of the whole procedure is jeopardized. Having administered sedation of various sorts for a number of different dentists one is very keenly aware of the enormous difference it makes to the ease of management of the sedation if injections are placed gently, painlessly and effectively. It is desirable to induce amnesia for the injection of local analgesic, but when diazepam is used as a sole agent for sedation, it is difficult at the time of giving of injections, to ensure that this will be so. Only a good deal of experience of the method, with careful follow up, will establish for a dentist a sound basis for estimating, at the time of a procedure, what is the degree of amnesia which may be expected. It is important to recognize of course that however desirable it may be, complete amnesia is not vital to the success of sedation procedures. When a patient remembers something of the treatment and is unworried by it, this may be of therapeutic value in overcoming his fears and in paving the way for acceptance of treatment in future with no sedation, or with a much less deep sedation. Amnesia can sometimes create minor difficulties with a second or subsequent treatment as when a patient protests, at the placement of injections "You did not do this last time". A kindly reminder that the patient does not really know what was done, followed by a gentle resumption of the procedure, will usually overcome this hurdle.

In healthy patients, if a dosage limit such as 0·2 mg per kilogram body weight be observed when using intravenous diazepam, results will usually be satisfactory and a useful period of sedation will be achieved. If, however, the sedation is inadequate or if it becomes inadequate after some 30 minutes, the question arises of giving a further dose. Only experience will give a sound basis for decision, but a few points relative to pharmacology may be made which will sub-stantially assist in deciding on a course of action.

Consider first the case in which the initial dose of diazepam appears to have been inadequate. The most important single consideration if overdose or an unnecessarily large dose is to be avoided, is that sufficient time be allowed for full effect of the primary dose to be apparent. Some ten minutes should elapse, and for most of this time the patient should be supine, comfortable and undisturbed: the dentist should consider three questions:

1. *Is the dose adequate?*

    If it is, the patient who is allowed to be undisturbed will usually be apt to drop off to sleep, at least for short periods. If the patient remains awake and alert this suggests inadequacy of dosage.

2. *If the dosage was inadequate, will a further dose help?*

    The answer to this should be sought along two lines. Firstly, is there a reason to suspect that this patient may need a higher dose, whether for reasons of physical robustness, a tendency to hyper-activity or to extreme anxiety. Secondly, has the drug had at least some effect in diminishing obvious manifestations of anxiety, for if it has some effect, then a further small dose will almost certainly be beneficial.

3. *What should be the size of a further dose?*

    The maximum should be one half of what has already been given. It should be given by slow increments watching for its effect. Not infrequently a quite small addition, for example, one quarter or one third of the initial dose will prove to be quite adequate. In the case in which inadequacy of sedation is manifest after one half to three quarters of an hour of operation, even more reservations must be made concerning the administration of further doses of diazepam. The beginner would be wise to curtail the operation, if improvement cannot be obtained by simple measures such as a brief respite from treatment, gentle reassurance or change of position in the chair. If the decision is made to give further diazepam at a late stage of the procedure, two essentials are that the dose be small, not more than half what has already been given, and that it be recognized that its effect can be expected to be rather prolonged. It is the prolongation of effect seen after unduly large doses of diazepam which tended to bring the drug into some disrepute, until this feature of its pharmacology was fully recognized. At the time of giving, further doses beyond that which induces adequate sedation seem to have very little effect. It is because of this feature, more than any other, that the need to keep a mental check on total dosage in any one session has been emphasized.

Combined techniques

The outstanding advantage of diazepam as a sedative in dentistry is the fact that extremely satisfactory sedation can usually be achieved with injection of a single drug. Its limitations have been noted, but these are slight in contrast to its tremendous potential for achieving satisfactory sedation. The need for repetitive administration in one session is almost nil. Where one person is to give sedation and carry out dental treatment there is greatest safety inherent in a method where the two tasks are performed in two quite distinct phases. Further, the potential of a method for undesirable complications is minimal if there are only the effects of a single agent to consider. Nevertheless, for the patient who demands or whose condition demands a greater degree of control over amnesia, but whose state also makes it desirable to avoid the unduly prolonged effects from high dosage diazepam, a great advantage can be obtained by judicious combination of diazepam and methohexitone sodium.

Diazepam is administered first in just the manner described above, but may be given in somewhat smaller dosage, then at a point where deeper sedation and a greater certainty of amnesic effect is wanted, a small dose of methohexitone is given. It is important to note the term 'small dose': the exact size will be found by trial, but the trial dose in an adult would be of the order of 5 or 10 mg. In combination with diazepam even this small dose may actually induce unconsciousness, and its effect will be far more prolonged than is usual. It also induces marked amnesia which extends to cover events which occurred before its administration, and to which the patient may have shown quite marked objection.

The retrograde amnesia induced by incremental doses of methohexitone has for some time been recognized by dentists who use sedation: it has been demonstrated experimentally in rats (Pearlman *et al* 1961) in relation to similar drugs. It can be used to advantage in the process of placing local analgesic injections, in the following manner: a dose of diazepam is given which will induce relaxation but is sufficiently small for awareness and co-operation to be fully present. Injection of local analgesic solution is then made. The patient is likely to register distaste, but will probably be able to co-operate. Immediately the injection is finished, a small dose of methohexitone is administered. It is likely that no further methohexitone will be needed for some time, little more for satisfactory sedation for the entire procedure, but amnesia for the local analgesic injection will be complete.

The combination of the different effects of diazepam and methohexitone in this way is a most satisfactory procedure, in the hands of the expert it gives extremely satisfactory results. It is most important, however, to emphasize its very different nature from use of diazepam alone, relative to inherent safety. As soon as incremental dosage of an agent such as methohexitone is used, the whole character of the procedure changes because, as set out in some detail in Chapter 7, the judgment of incremental dosage is a matter of extreme difficulty. With the best intentions in the world it is fatally easy to push the patient into a state of deep anaesthesia. If the person giving the drug is competent in the field of airway maintenance and intermittent positive pressure breathing, this is of little significance, but the average dentist is not, and this type of technique is not for him.

The question of education in anaesthetic methods which a dentist needs if he is to carry out sedation techniques safely, has been touched upon. It will be dealt with further in the next chapter, but one important point must be made here. It is frequently implied, if not stated explicitly, that the dentist who learns the technique of intravenous sedation using diazepam can, after applying this successfully to increasing numbers of patients in his practice, graduate to the use of more complex techniques, of which additional use of incremental methohexitone is often quoted as an example. This view point is largely fallacious. After using diazepam in practice, the dentist will have gained experience in administration of one intravenous sedative agent, and in performing dental work on the supine sedated patient—and nothing more. He will have the technical skill necessary to give methohexitone, but may lack entirely the skills necessary to get out of serious trouble, into which he can land with the greatest facility.

He may well be regarded as having a reasonable basis upon which to undergo further training, but this training, to be in any wise adequate for safety in management of other forms of sedation, would emphatically need to involve an extended period carrying out practical procedures in the anaesthetic department of a hospital. Only in this context can anything but the simplest of methods of dental sedation be regarded in any sense as 'safe'.

CHAPTER 10
COMPLICATIONS OF SEDATION

There is a dearth of reliable information concerning complications of dental sedation procedures. The mortality is extremely low and serious complications are certainly uncommon, but this could well be the result merely of the good general health of the vast majority of patients and of the low morbidity inherent in the surgery. Death has occasionally resulted from a dental sedation procedure (Bourne 1970): to regard such an incident as being a unique event among many thousands of cases in which there is no vestige of trouble seems to be a slightly unrealistic attitude: yet to obtain first-hand information about the circumstances which obtain when the solo dental practitioner administers sedation in his surgery with the assistance only of his nurses is hardly feasible. The mere presence of an anaesthetist observing such a situation may tend to alter its character completely. It is therefore necessary to seek information from a variety of sources and attempt integration of this in the framework of the anaesthetist's background knowledge.

THE ANAESTHETIST'S VIEW

Anaesthetists probably take an unduly pessimistic view of dental sedation procedures, especially those in which barbiturates are given intravenously. Outspoken criticism by anaesthetists reflects a view which seems to be negated by undeniable evidence of the safety of the procedures in the hands of many dentists. The reason is that the anaesthetist overlooks important differences which usually exist between dental sedation procedures and the procedures of general anaesthesia. They are differences of degree rather than of kind, but when coupled with the usually good general health of dental patients are sufficient to account for the remarkable way in which the dentist with very little grounding in anaesthetic procedures can have such an apparently high success rate in dental sedation.

The surgery with which the anaesthetist is usually involved demands a much deeper plane of depression of consciousness than is ever desirable or indeed usual in dental sedation. The dentist does no more than diminish patient response, he certainly should not attempt to abolish response solely by use of depressant drugs. The levels of sedation employed in the dental surgery are very much lighter than those which the anaesthetist is accustomed to use, and therefore inherently less dangerous.

The dentist usually employs one sedative agent, occasionally more. It is not usual for the patient to receive any narcotic analgesic such as pethidine or morphine: when these drugs are used in dental sedation it will be in very low dose. The majority of the patients with whom the anaesthetist deals in connection with surgical procedures have, for one reason or another, received a narcotic in effective dosage. These drugs have a most significant depressant action on the respiratory drive and thereby aggravate the severity of the effects of obstruction to respiration in the case of laryngospasm. The healthy patient who is moderately sedated with methohexitone or diazepam or even with a combination of these still retains, as a rule, a lively ability to respond effectively to minor degrees of respiratory obstruction and to overcome them by his own efforts with minimal aid.

As an additional factor precipitating laryngospasm, the anaesthetist has the irritant effects of volatile anaesthetic agents to reckon with in many cases. The dentist does not use these and is free from this annoyance. He is faced by a different potential cause of laryngospasm: the risk of contamination of the pharynx by water or blood or other foreign material dropping back from the mouth. The dentist has this area under observation, however, and by vigilance in the use of suction and mouth packing can generally keep the pharynx free of contamination. These few comments on differences between anaesthetic practice and sedation may help the anaesthetist to understand the lower complication rate apparent in the dentist's procedures. He needs also to understand something of the motivation and attitude of the dentist who carries out sedation. If he is to be in a position to advise and help the dentist it is most necessary that the anaesthetist have some understanding of the background of the dentist.

THE DENTIST'S VIEW

The dentist who uses sedation does so because of a keen awareness of a need for it. He is conscious of the deficiencies of local analgesia, some of which are noted in Chapter 7 (page 98), his desire to provide his patient with a degree of sedation sufficient to ameliorate these is understandable and indeed laudable. The dentist does not have training and experience in management of airway and other problems which the anaesthetist possesses and is aware of this relative deficiency in his education. He tries to compensate by a strong determination to keep out of trouble. This determination is reinforced by his mentors—their writings reflect it—and sometimes in a fashion which antagonizes the anaesthetist when he tries to learn about intravenous sedation by reading books. Such texts are written, in many instances, by a dentist who is an experienced practical anaesthetist. He has usually gained an almost intuitive knowledge of respiratory problems and has a great deal of skill in their management. In an effort to inculcate safe practice, his writings attribute his success and his remarkable freedom from complications to rigid following of set rituals, to close observation of the patient and to perfection in performance of, for example, placement of mouth packs to protect the pharynx. It is appropriate to quote here the doyen of intravenous dentists, Drummond Jackson (1971a). He says in his account of his technique: "... intermittent methohexitone is the finest of all intravenous techniques for the conscientious expert—but quite impossible for the 80 per cent man ... ". The evident implication is that the placing of moistened cellulose-sponge flange packs to protect the pharynx in the sedated patient can and must be always carried out with absolute perfection. It seems also to be implied that occurrence of laryngospasm strongly suggests carelessness in packing. The intention is plain—to encourage those who use the technique to aspire to ever greater heights of perfection. In those who lack the experience and remarkable dexterity, knowledge and skill of their mentor and who are trying to use this technique in a dental practice, one feels that such teaching may engender a different attitude. It may make the dentist close his eyes to troubles and make him unwilling to acknowledge his problems or to report them. He will find that the healthy patient will usually 'get by' even if there are minor degrees of laryngospasm, to report it would be an admission of carelessness—better to keep quiet. The average man can only feel a deep sense of inadequacy when he compares his complication rate with the published results of his mentor's first 40,000 cases (Drummond Jackson, 1962) which demonstrate a uniquely low incidence of complications.

THE BALANCED VIEW

The empirical teaching in dental texts on sedation which places emphasis on 'keeping out of trouble', is comprehensible when consideration is given to the person to whom they are chiefly directed. It is often the post-graduate dentist who is attempting to use sedation after a very brief course of instruction. Soundness in recognition of minor complications and in their management cannot be taught briefly and cannot be learned from books. Active intervention in cases of minor spasm in the lightly sedated patient may cause more trouble than would result from allowing the patient to overcome the problem spontaneously. There is something to be said, therefore, for putting stress, in these circumstances, on positive avoidance of difficulties and giving little mention to respiratory and circulatory problems unless they present with such severity as to demand action: and the dentist has usually been well taught in regard to these emergency situations.

Where dentists are to undergo a longer period of teaching and clinical experience in sedation, it is reasonable to take a different attitude and to go much more fully into recognition and active management of respiratory problems in particular. It is natural that this aspect of sedation should be taught in conjunction with the practice of general anaesthesia, in which there is a greater incidence of problems and where the generally greater depth of anaesthesia makes active measures more applicable. The importance of this teaching for dental undergraduate and graduate students has received emphasis in Part II and the dentists who have learned some of the skills of the anaesthetist will be very well equipped for the safe performance of sedation. The incidence and nature of complications in sedation is very different from that of general anaesthesia, so it is important that knowledge gained in the practice of anaesthesia be tempered by a realistic awareness of the different nature of sedation. For this reason an attempt is now made to examine precisely what

are the complications liable to occur in sedation, and in what circumstances they may be serious, so that the dentist may be best equipped
to recognize the risks and take effective steps to avoid or to deal with
the problems.

THE MODE OF OCCURRENCE OF PROBLEMS

There is one uncommon but very significant cause of serious trouble
in the course of sedation which has been well documented (Bourne
1957, 1973), namely the upright or reclining position in the dental
chair which may make hypotension resulting from a fainting attack
or other causes have very serious consequences (see Chapter 3, page
30). To avoid this, the ideal is to have the patient horizontal. As the
patient who needs sedation may be nervous and may dislike the
sensation of lying flat, it is common practice to compromise and have
the head end and back of the chair slightly raised (Foreman 1972). It
is important that the legs be raised to a horizontal position or higher,
also that the dangers inherent in the position be recognized. Patients
should be placed horizontal as soon as they will accept the position.
It is necessary to be able to place the patient quickly in the 'head low'
position in case of emergency, and a limitation of some modern
chairs in this regard needs to be noted. The reclining chair with
electrically operated movements may take a significant period for the
back to move down into this position. It is an advantage in these
cases to have a chair which has, in addition to the electrically controlled movement, a pedal which when pressed allows the whole
chair to move 'see-saw' fashion. Such a chair can be speedily moved
from reclining to 'head low' position.

Apart from this primary circulatory collapse, it is to be expected
that airway obstruction will be the common starting point for serious
trouble. Laryngospasm will be taken as the example, dealing with its
recognition and management, and the circumstances in which it may
lead to problems.

Laryngospasm

It is of particular importance in light sedation that the significance of
laryngospasm as a protective reflex be kept in mind. If this is done, it
is easy to manage the minor degrees which occur under these con-

ditions. There may be brief stridor, or there may be a virtually silent catch in the breath. One should immediately look to the packing and the pharynx and remove the pack while using the sucker gently to remove any mucus and to prevent any material from falling back. The state of consciousness or depth of sedation is determined by response to touching the fauces or soft palate with the sucker: gagging or swallowing indicate a light state of sedation, it may be confidently expected that, if the mandible is gently supported to prevent pharyngeal obstruction, the patient will shortly resume normal respiration, perhaps after a swallow or cough. When managed in this way laryngospasm under light sedation is no more than a momentary interruption. Only if there is failure of quick recovery or persisting stridor should the next stage of treatment be needed.

When a patient develops laryngeal stridor, packs should be removed and suction instituted as mentioned. Despite these measures stridor may persist or worsen, or a complete obstruction may develop with the patient making vigorous efforts to overcome it. There will sometimes be a severe, generalized restlessness which is characteristic of oxygen lack. The correct treatment in this case is that, after adequate suction to clear mouth and pharynx, a face mask should be applied and intermittent positive pressure breathing carried out— preferably with oxygen: failing this, with air from a recoil bag resuscitator. The pressure on the bag should be gently sustained until a movement of the patient allows some oxygen in: it is a case of 'persuading' oxygen past the glottis and ensuring that any small inspiratory effort is assisted.

Patients who develop laryngospasm which persists in the manner described will almost invariably recover, even without any active treatment—if helped by jaw support and perhaps turned on one side. It is worth while to consider briefly what may be the circumstances in which spontaneous recovery may not occur, and one such factor is anything which allows aspiration of foreign material to irritate or to obstruct the glottis. The importance of removing packs and using the sucker has been stressed: the other source of trouble is occurrence of vomiting or regurgitation of stomach contents. The presence in the pharynx of acid gastric juice may prolong laryngospasm: if any is aspirated past the glottis it may induce a severe pulmonary oedema. If there is solid food in the stomach, it may impact in the larynx. This will be a serious situation, yet it is one from which a healthy patient may well emerge unscathed with minimal assistance. It is probable that serious consequences are unlikely to arise unless the patient was suffering from some pre-existing disease unknown to the dentist.

The patient with pre-existing disease

The process of overcoming airway obstruction unaided places a considerable stress on the cardiovascular system. As soon as obstruction to breathing occurs, the failure of pulmonary ventilation leads to hypoxaemia—diminution of the oxygen partial pressure in the arterial blood—and elevation of the level of carbon dioxide. These are the factors which lead to the increased respiratory drive which usually overcomes the obstruction, but they are detrimental to the patient who has any cardiovascular disease. The respiratory efforts against obstruction place a further load on the circulation, and there is also secretion of catechol-amines with additional adverse effects. These then are the circumstances in which a fatal outcome is likely. Because its occurrence requires the coincidental happening of several events, it will be rare in any conditions. It is nonetheless important to consider how it may be prevented, and there are evidently three aspects to be examined.

1. Airway maintenance:

Where obstruction to breathing is always recognized promptly and treated actively there will be little likelihood of serious trouble. If the patient never exerts a strong respiratory effort against obstruction, the problems of aspiration or of cardiovascular collapse will not materialize. It is of very great importance that dentists undertaking sedation be thoroughly schooled in all aspects of airway maintenance and protection.

2. Aspiration risks:

The aspiration of vomitus is familiar to anaesthetists as being a frequent factor in anaesthetic fatalities. One is concerned to read of the casual dismissal by some authorities of any need for fasting in preparation for certain dental sedation procedures. It seems evident that widespread relaxation of a rule of fasting must be a factor in increasing potentially fatal incidents.

3. Pre-existing disease:

The patient with cardiovascular disease is likely to be unable to withstand stresses due to unrelieved airway obstruction. If such patients are to undergo sedation or general anaesthesia, this should be administered only by a skilled anaesthetist. The problems facing the dentist in relation to medical assessment of his patients have been mentioned, they are difficult of solution. It is important to recognize that care in this field should not stop at the pre-anaesthetic medical examination. The pre-operative assessment which the anaesthetist makes is essentially provisional and is checked by the patient's response to all features of the anaesthetic administration. Nor does the wise anaesthetist take liberties with any patient: he regards it as intolerable to allow respiratory obstruction or any interference with ventilation or oxygenation to persist, even in the healthy patient. Only with the application of these high standards by the physician anaesthetist can maximum safety be assured, but the conscientious dentist can do much for safety in sedation by attention to detail. The level of sedation will always be as light as possible to ensure that in the event of any airway or circulatory difficulties the patient will not be at a disadvantage from respiratory and circulatory depression. Attention to pre-operative fasting will be careful to minimize the risks of vomiting, and sedation will be kept light to minimize its incidence. He will question his patients carefully in an effort to ensure that significant pre-existing disease is not overlooked—he will always exercise care in selection of patients for sedation by himself and be prepared to call a consultant if needed.

ILL-ADVISED SELECTION OF PATIENTS

There is an unfortunate trend in patient selection advocated in certain texts on dental sedation—well exemplified by McCarthy (1972). In the introduction to a section on psychosedation, which describes inhalational and intravenous methods of sedation, the statement is made "Adequate pain/anxiety control is second only to a proper pre-treatment physical evaluation in the prevention of medical emergencies". A specific recommendation is made that the dentist who has a 'high-risk' patient to treat should employ intravenous sedation with diazepam or brief anaesthesia with unsupplemented intravenous methohexitone in the dental surgery. The term 'high-risk' patient is stated to include "patients with a history of cardiovascular disease, arterial hypertension and cerebrovascular disease, in whom endogenous epinephrine production in response to stress may result in dangerously elevated blood pressure and cardiac arrhythmias".

The suggestion that intravenous administration of cerebral depressants increases the *safety* of dental treatment with local analgesia in poor-risk patients is highly questionable. It seems that far too little cognizance is taken of the dangers of administration of potent depressant drugs by the intravenous route—to poor risk patients in particular.

Dosage of intravenous agents

Administration of an intravenous agent such as methohexitone or thiopentone may cause respiratory and circulatory depression. Respiratory depression in slight degree is a common observation, it is marked as a rule only if narcotic or other depressant premedication has been given. Respiratory depression is easily managed, it is serious only if there is concurrent obstruction to respiration. This may be treated, if not prevented, by early positive action, for example, application of a face mask and administration of oxygen by intermittent positive pressure. In most cases support of the mandible is all that is needed, the respiratory depression accompanies a corresponding fall in metabolism and no hypoxaemia usually results. The anaesthetist tends nevertheless to employ intermittent positive pressure breathing early, even if it is not intended to follow on with gaseous anaesthesia. The reason is the desire to forestall trouble, to never allow any suspicion of underventilation to persist, in case respiratory obstruction should arise unexpectedly. In the dentists' cases the lower dose and slower rate of injection, with the absence of depressant premedication, is responsible for a lower incidence of respiratory depression.

Circulatory depression is more potentially serious: it is seen in various degrees—most commonly there is some fall in blood pressure. This is usually minimal in healthy patients, if it is a small drop and the patient is horizontal there is no cause for alarm. A more serious degree of circulatory depression is manifest as a rule by a change of colour in the skin. Varying degrees of pallor and cyanosis cause a grey appearance—this needs prompt treatment: the legs should be raised a little to improve venous return and oxygen given with intermittent positive pressure. Any uncertainty about immediate restoration of satisfactory circulation should lead to urgent closed chest cardiac compression which is maintained until recovery is assured.

Severe circulatory collapse from this cause is a rare event in the hands of the capable anaesthetist because he will usually have been alerted by his findings on pre-operative examination if the patient's cardiovascular condition demands special care, and will be warned to avoid relative overdosage. It is necessary to stress that the dose which produces ill effects in the case of severe cardiovascular disease may be very small—much less than one half of a normal induction dose may suffice. In addition to a careful pre-operative examination to detect cases at risk, it is most desirable to employ always a mode of administration of intravenous agents which will test adequately the patient's response and give some protection against overdose.

Safe practice in intravenous anaesthesia

A suitable routine is that a 'test dose' of the drug is used in every case. An appropriate dose for an adult who is apparently healthy would be thiopentone 50–100 mg or methohexitone 20–40 mg according to size. The full effect of this should be seen and assessed before any further drug is given. Any further dose given is based upon body weight and response to the test dose. This method sounds simple and fool-proof, but attention needs to be drawn to its weaknesses, under three headings.

1. Circulation time from a vein in the arm to an artery in the brain is about 20 seconds normally, a drug given intravenously is seen to act in little more than that time. In cases of cardiovascular disease, especially if there is cardiac failure—a condition in which relative overdose is dangerous—there is usually prolongation of the circulation time, which fact can readily give the impression that the test dose has had little or no effect. The anaesthetist who has examined his patient will usually be forewarned and wait to see the delayed action, noting the prolonged circulation time as being a significant diagnostic finding. If the dentist overlooks this he is likely to give a further dose which may be dangerous.

2. Advantages of quick injection: as the dentist gains experience in giving methohexitone to patients for brief procedures he learns the advantages to be gained by a fairly rapid rate of injection of solution (Drummond Jackson, 1971b) in that it controls the

patient well, permits a smaller total dose and generally provides a
a more satisfactory anaesthesia. The use of a test dose diminishes
the efficacy of this method and may be omitted on that account.

3. Observations made after the test dose: Few anaesthetists will
look for signs of circulatory depression after a test dose. One
usually looks only for its effect on consciousness, perhaps on
respiration. The application of this test may therefore be completely misleading in the case of a patient who has a high tolerance
to methohexitone engendered by alcohol intake but also has a
cardiac lesion—aortic stenosis, for example—which limits
increase of cardiac output in response to the vasodilatation due to
methohexitone.

This is a weakness of such a test—this and the usually negative
results when it is applied to healthy patients tend to make even the
conscientious dentist apply it in somewhat desultory fashion. Nor
are dentists alone in this: the rarity of undue sensitivity to the action
of intravenous drugs in the absence of fairly plain clinical warning
means that the anaesthetist may easily believe for a long period that
he is using a safe technique—until disillusionment suddenly comes.

There is no easy solution to this dilemma, either for the anaesthetist
or for the dentist using sedation. Both need always to be on the alert
to detect pre-existing disease and to be especially cautious in administration of drugs in these cases. It is necessary always to be fully
prepared to handle the worst result that can stem from relative
overdose—namely circulatory arrest.

PART IV

PROBLEMS

Consideration of general anaesthesia for dentistry has in the past been mostly confined to out-patient practice, with emphasis on selection of patients who are in good health. It has not been usual to consider the problems of the poor risk patient in this context. An attempt is therefore made to provide some guidelines to assist the specialist anaesthetist in the management of these cases.

Those who teach dental undergraduates feel at a loss to know what will be the future pattern of practice in relation to application of sedation procedures in dentistry. There is no place here for pontifical statements about 'who should or should not do what', but there is a need for examination in depth of the requirements of dental practice in this regard. There is a still greater need to understand the current limitations of specialist anaesthetist training in the dental field, as well as the limitations of dental teaching in the fields of clinical medicine and general anaesthesia.

These are a few of the reasons for the presumptuous title of the final chapter, which attempts a review of some of these factors.

CHAPTER 11
POOR RISK PATIENTS

Patients may be regarded as a 'poor risk' for general anaesthesia by virtue of their medical condition, or their surgical condition, or a combination of these. In the past the tendency has been in dental anaesthesia to select only healthy patients for general anaesthesia and to relegate all less good risk patients for the dentist to manage unassisted with local analgesia. One consequence of this is that the anaesthetist who has worked in these conditions will be of little help to the dentist in relation to problem cases in which he is not prepared to administer general anaesthesia. When one is aware of the extreme dislike, even terror of dental treatment which some patients manifest, one listens with more sympathy to the patient who seeks general anaesthesia but in whom it is felt to carry an unreasonable risk, and one is prepared to consider a combination of local analgesia with carefully administered sedation as an alternative to endotracheal general anaesthesia.

It is in this field even more than in the case of the healthy patient, that emphasis is needed on 'patient handling', at least as much as on agents used to induce sedation. If an older patient is merely allowed to rest supine for a period before and after some extractions are carefully performed with local analgesia, acceptance of the procedure is likely to be good and complications minimal. Sedation of any sort should be cautiously employed only as a supplement to such considerate gentle management.

When first requested to assist with this type of case the anaesthetist may be at a loss to know how best to proceed; some general advice is therefore given which is based on experience. For the patient who is to be a day patient in a ward, it is sometimes convenient to order a premedication to be given by the nursing staff by intramuscular injection. This may be given some time—an hour or more—before the procedure, and the aim is merely to induce tranquillity. A suitable choice of drugs is pethidine with atropine, but the anaesthetist will use drugs with which he is familiar. Doses should in any case be much smaller than those generally employed for pre-anaesthetic medication in general surgery. Pethidine will be given in a dose of about one half milligram per kilogram body weight, its effect is not needed as an analgesic, this combined perhaps with promethazine 10 mg will induce a sufficient degree of sedation as a rule. Atropine 0·5 mg may be given to diminish the likelihood of fainting and assist the surgeon by drying oral secretion. The anaesthetist should be present at least at the start of the surgical procedure, and may administer a small dose of diazepam by the intravenous route. The patient who is premedicated is more susceptible to its respiratory depressant effects, the dose should be small and cautiously given. The surgeon then places local analgesic injections, allows them some time to act and proceeds to surgery. He should use appropriate mouth packing, as described in Chapter 3 to protect the airway from soiling.

It is reasonable to question in what way such a procedure as this is safer than endotracheal general anaesthesia. The answer depends on several considerations.

THE DECISION FOR ANAESTHESIA OR SEDATION

A basic risk of general anaesthesia is respiratory and circulatory depression from the drugs used. In performing sedation, the anaesthetist may so choose his agents and give them in such small dose that significant depression can be avoided and yet the patient rendered comfortable and quite often amnesic.

Airway protection by an endotracheal tube is complete while the tube is correctly placed, but its introduction requires profound muscular relaxation by anaesthesia and neuromuscular blockade. When sedation is used without a tube, airway protection is largely in the hands of the surgeon. It is necessary to give due consideration to the nature of the surgery—the number and placement of the teeth as as well as the expected difficulty of removal—before a decision is made on this aspect of the case.

When a surgeon and an anaesthetist have worked together on many cases, sound decisions can readily be made. The surgeon will know something of the problems which may be expected from an endotracheal general anaesthetic, the anaesthetist will likewise be able to anticipate what conditions would be like under sedation. The cardinal feature deserves emphasis once more. Sedation must be no more than a light supplement for skilful, gentle work under local analgesia. If there is any suggestion of increasing the dose of sedative drugs to cover deficiencies of local analgesia, the procedure loses its safety. The anaesthetist who learns the sound practice of this type of procedure in the dental school has learned something which will be of general utility. For patients who are not in a good risk category, who are undergoing surgery which can be performed with local analgesia, the use of judiciously applied sedation will be of the utmost value. With these patients however, as with dental cases, the importance of careful handling is paramount: there are few better places than dental practice in which to become familiar with this art.

CONSERVATIVE DENTAL TREATMENT

General anaesthesia for conservation of teeth—for the performance of restorative dental treatment—is resorted to when a patient requires such therapy but its performance with local analgesia is not feasible. Some normal adults elect to have their dentistry done in this way: apart from these there are two main groups for whom it is undertaken.

Children whose co-operation can not be obtained constitute one group, the extent of which depends, of course, on the ability of the dentist to succeed in the face of opposition. The procedures may be prolonged, in which case the anaesthetic should be endotracheal. This carries risks in children which are greatest in the very young. It is most desirable that any sound alternative be considered and tried if possible to avoid the need for general anaesthesia, and that if this be needed, it be given by an anaesthetist who is skilled at endotracheal intubation in children.

The other major group of patients comprises those who are mentally retarded or afflicted with cerebral palsy or other brain damage and cannot co-operate on this account. The general condition of some of these patients may be such as to cause some concern about general anaesthesia. The anaesthetist will be assisted in making decisions about their management if he has some appreciation of the basis of the dentistry to be performed, of the motivation in attempting conservation rather than extraction of carious teeth.

The patient who is retarded or spastic is not likely to be able to manage dentures, therefore his natural teeth should be conserved if possible. Oral hygiene in these patients may be poor, however, and even the best restorative dentistry may therefore be short lived in its effect. It is helpful if decisions on the scope of dental treatment for these patients be guided by a dentist who has sufficient experience to make a realistic assessment of the prospect and to keep conservative work within reasonable bounds. The dentist who knows that his patient is unapproachable unless asleep may feel obliged to make his work as complete and as perfect as possible, and tend to make the procedure dangerously long. The knowledge that the surgery is essentially elective heightens a keen desire on the part of the anaesthetist to keep the whole procedure free from risk. A source of danger in the patient who is not normal is the increased risk associated with a prolonged anaesthetic. The dentist cannot, as a rule, give in advance a reliable estimate of the duration of the operation, any more than the anaesthetist can say before induction that any particular duration of anaesthesia is safe. It is important that dentist and anaesthetist be able to reach agreement, therefore this simple scheme is recommended.

The dentist, in planning his restorations, should divide the work into two sections which may be expected to occupy equal length of time. He should proceed with the first segment and a short time before completing it inform the anaesthetist that he is approaching the half-way mark in the total procedure. By this stage the anaesthetist knows how his patient is responding to the situation. He should not find it difficult to decide whether, in the circumstances which obtain, it is reasonable to maintain anaesthesia for as long again to allow completion of the whole of the work, or whether it would be wiser to terminate the procedure shortly and finish the work on another day. This concept is worthwhile in any circumstances, but particularly when anaesthesia is undertaken in the dentist's rooms. It is a simple means of avoiding misunderstandings in which either the dentist feels that he is not getting a fair deal or the anaesthetist feels that he is being imposed upon to the detriment of his patient.

MANAGEMENT OF DISABLED PATIENTS

For many reasons, these patients can often not be seen in advance by the anaesthetist, there is usually a need to make a quick assessment of the prospect in relation to general anaesthesia, certain points are particularly relevant. In the case of any patient who is bed-ridden or predominantly immobile, enquiry about the patient's eating habits is worthwhile: can he chew and swallow, does he tend to choke on his food? Enquiry should also be made as to whether there have been recurring episodes of chest trouble. The answers convey some idea of the efficacy of protective reflexes: if these are not fairly sound, then any anaesthesia is hazardous, but prolonged or deep anaesthesia should certainly not be undertaken.

The possibility of anaemia should be borne in mind and a haemo-globin estimation performed if indicated. Upper respiratory infection is hard to assess: nasal catarrh may be persistent, and one may need to ask a reliable relative whether the discharge is more copious or more purulent than is usual. It is important to keep continually in mind the feasibility of terminating the operative procedure at short notice if the anaesthetic is not satisfactory: this is a safety feature of dental work as noted in Chapter 3 (page 52). Should laryngoscopy and intubation reveal, for example, an unduly large amount of mucopus in the trachea, one would be inclined to clear this and then terminate the procedure as soon as possible.

Cases of Down's syndrome demand caution on several counts. Congenital malformation of the heart is not uncommon and should be looked for. Difficulty with intubation may arise not only from general configuration but particularly from the excessive lymphoid tissue which is usually present in the pharynx. This tissue may affect the back of the tongue in particular, there may be virtual obliteration of the vallecula by tissue which bleeds freely when touched by the laryngoscope. Adult cases are often obese, which further increases anaesthetic difficulties. Monitoring during anaesthesia of such in-active patients frequently shows a low blood pressure—70 or 80 mmHg systolic is common. Experience suggests that this is harmless, and that more notice should be taken of adequacy of perfusion as indicated by a satisfactory peripheral circulation. Endotracheal anaesthesia is the rule for conservative dentistry, exception should be made only where the work is to be extremely brief and where intubation is strongly contra-indicated.

In relation to the question of a prolonged general anaesthetic for a normal adult to have extensive restoration of teeth—one can only express the hope that in the future dentists will make increasing use of sedation to supplement local analgesia for such patients. The anaesthetist finds these procedures tedious and exacting: the dentist usually prefers to carry out the work in his own surgery rather than in hospital. Conditions for anaesthesia and recovery may be less than ideal unless the dental office is unusually spacious and well equipped. An anaesthetic which is prolonged beyond an hour or so inevitably carries increased risk of complications—in general, careful light sedation or relative analgesia would be safer for the patient.

SURGICAL PROBLEMS

Patients who are in good general health may present an increased risk in relation to general anaesthesia because of their surgical condition. A common example in dentistry is found in the patient who presents with an acute infection as a result of a neglected dental condition— with cellulitis or abscess.

The anaesthetist in the dental school will be asked from time to time to administer a general anaesthetic for such cases—sometimes with some urgency. He will be better able to manage the case if he is acquainted with the surgical problem. In the course of his pre-anaesthetic examination, the anaesthetist should seek out certain features. If there is swelling of the face the history is important: how long has it been present? Has any antibiotic been given? What has been the response? Has there been a similar swelling before which has been reduced by antibiotic administration but has recurred? Examination should carefully delineate the extent of swelling, in the case of the lower jaw for example, bimanual palpation of the floor of the mouth should be undertaken. With cellulitis in relation to an upper tooth, swelling of the soft palate or pharynx should be looked for. The possibility of airway obstruction should be borne in mind, and any sign of trismus, of limitation of jaw opening, is of special significance. These are cases in which fasting in preparation for general anaesthesia is of special importance, as swelling or trismus may accentuate airway problems and there may be a risk of rupture of an abscess into mouth or pharynx. The anaesthetist should take an interest in surgical management of these cases and try to ensure that those responsible have in mind at every stage the possible need for general anaesthesia so that the patient will be requested to present fasting on any occasion when this may be necessary.

Apart from the question of fasting, limitation of jaw opening is the major cause for concern in these cases and deserves some comment.

Trismus

The importance of looking for this in dental cases has been stressed and the significance of the history mentioned. This may give a clue to the likely effect of general anaesthesia and neuromuscular blockade on the degree of jaw opening. In the case of bony trismus—that due to some zygomatic fractures or to malunited fracture in the region of the temporomandibular joint, there may be no increase in opening. Trismus associated with acute infection of recent onset may be expected to relax completely. Caution is needed in longer standing infection, especially if treatment with antibiotic has been previously given but definitive treatment of the offending tooth neglected— usually by patient default. The resultant woody swelling, with the apt colloquial name of 'antibioma' may be associated with a particularly unyielding trismus and be difficult of management from every point of view.

The conduct of the anaesthetic is a technical problem for the anaesthetist: it is usually capable of solution if it is recognized in advance. The anaesthetist who elects to perform blind nasal intubation in a case of 'set' trismus should answer just one question before starting: 'What exactly will I do if I cannot pass the tube blindly?' The approach should be planned with care, full use should be made of measures such as pre-oxygenation and nasal vasoconstrictors. The plan needs to cover every eventuality and be so carried out that in the unlikely event of tracheostomy being required it may be done as a deliberate rather than a hasty procedure.

CHAPTER 12
THE FUTURE

The application of clinical anaesthesia to dentistry has thus far been examined chiefly in the context of the Dental School. The plan described in Chapter 6 effects a compromise between the ideal and the feasible in the out-patient clinic. Outside the school, there is a variety of practice in the Dental Surgery or office. Traditional 'nasal gas' may be given by dentist or doctor, or the specialist anaesthetist may use endotracheal intubation. The dentist may employ various types of sedation with or without local analgesia. It is essential to examine the training and education of the various people involved, to look closely at criticisms which are made of their practices, and thereby to formulate a workable scheme for future teaching and practice, in an endeavour to realize the optimism implicit in the title of this chapter.

Specialist anaesthetists give voice to a wide range of opinions in relation to administration of general anaesthesia by dentists. These vary from apparent acceptance (e.g., Galley 1974) to the absolute disapproval shown by many specialists in the United Kingdom, the North American continent, Australia and elsewhere. These contrasting views are perhaps comprehensible when considered in relation to the rapid development which has taken place in the field of anaesthesia. The senior anaesthetist will, in the past, have known dentists who were most capable in techniques of anaesthesia and whose knowledge all round approached that of the medical anaesthetists of their day. Steady progress in integration of medicine and physiology with clinical anaesthesia however renders the classical practices of dental anaesthesia ever more anachronistic, and the need for complete re-appraisal more urgent. Sedation, moreover, is an entirely new concept to the anaesthetist: its safety cannot be assessed by those whose knowledge is confined to general anaesthesia. Only a physician-anaesthetist with experience of all types of general anaesthesia for dentistry and of sedation—both administering it himself and seeing dentists use it—can have any concept of the true safety of sedation, only he can formulate any idea of what type of education and undergraduate training and experience may be appropriate for the dentist who is to undertake sedation in private practice.

CURRENT UNDERGRADUATE TEACHING

Teaching in general anaesthesia currently given to undergraduates in many Dental Schools does not provide a sound basis for post-graduate study or practice of sedation. Treating anaesthesia as being essentially a technical skill is inadequate, further, the manner of teaching has tended to mislead the undergraduate in regard to his own capabilities and technical competence. Those who teach in the Dental School have tended to perpetuate the idea of a simple method of anaesthesia which is universally applicable, but this air of simplicity has too often been largely spurious. It conceals the fact that a considerable degree of skill and much experience are needed for consistently good results in such procedures. Perhaps in the past this has represented a harmless deception, for the graduating dentist would likely move out into a practice where nasal nitrous oxide was a standard technique, and he would learn the art by using it under supervision. If however he moves out into a practice where sedation—or intermittent anaesthesia—with intravenous methohexitone (Brietal-Lilly) is the rule, his undergraduate instruction will be of little use—indeed it may prove to be quite misleading. He will have been taught maintenance of a clear airway, recognition of obstruction and methods of dealing with it. Such knowledge gained in the context of light gas anaesthesia will have little relevance in the patient whose breathing is quiet as a result of the depressant effect of an intravenous barbiturate. In such a case laryngospasm may develop silently and be difficult of recognition, intermittent positive pressure breathing with a face mask should be readily resorted to if the patient is not to be allowed to slip into a parlous state from hypoxia (Chapter 10, page 143).

The burgeoning practice of intravenous sedation by graduate dentists suggests that, in the short instructional courses at which they so often 'learn to do it', the practice of sedation is likewise presented as a simple technical exercise. They may fail to realize that the 'success' of their subsequent practice most likely depends on ignoring minor problems and placing reliance upon the robustness of the healthy human in resisting asphyxiation. Sedation can be taught more soundly, and it must be. The necessary pre-requisite is establishment in the Dental School of sound practice and teaching of general anaesthesia. As a result there tends to be less overwhelming pressure for the use of sedation and better opportunities for its restrained development.

Sedation has too often developed as a result of the default of general anaesthesia. The limitations of sedation, including poor conditions for dentistry, have been tolerated because nothing better was available. The fuller incorporation of the anaesthetist-in-training into the teaching practice of the dental school will be beneficial, for when he gains much of his practice in basic techniques in this environment, he will come to respect it. He will understand the requirements and problems of dentistry and will have opportunities to see dentists employing sedation and to establish with them a degree of rapport which has in the past been all too rare.

These changes will affect the dentist also. He has too often put up with mediocre conditions for dentistry because of deficiencies in anaesthesia or sedation. After some experience of first class anaesthesia he is less willing to put up with a squirming, groaning, unco-operative patient, as is sometimes the case when unsupplemented intravenous agents are used. It will no longer be sufficient justification that dentistry is performed which might have been impossible otherwise, and that the patient survives and thinks it is wonderful! The standards by which procedures are judged become inevitably more critical.

THE ANAESTHETIST IN THE DENTAL SURGERY

Although one might feel that the specialist anaesthetist would be the best person to handle anaesthesia in the dentist's surgery, this is not necessarily the case: many factors militate against success of such a practice and one needs to look at them fully. His most pressing handicap may be summed up in one word—diffidence. He is apt to feel that he should not be there. There has been, up to the present, no adequate, authoritative teaching which explicitly relates dental anaesthesia to the rest of the specialty: the anaesthetist is at a loss to know what is the best mode of management of cases. If the dentist and his staff have been accustomed to handling large numbers of general anaesthetic cases, the anaesthetist may hesitate to take definitive steps to alter their practices even when these seem to him to be very wrong—for example, having the patient sitting up in the chair.

There is much evidence which suggests that general anaesthesia in the dental surgery is less safe than is sedation administered by dentists. The realistic attitude for example of professional liability insurers in the U.S.A. seems to be quite definite on this point. The anaesthesiologist's premium is quite considerable—there is a significant mortality from general anaesthesia in the dental 'office', and it is increasingly difficult to find anyone who will defend the practice in court. Yet the same insurers apparently see no reason to use financial sanctions to discourage the practice of sedation by dentists (Trieger 1972). Figures from a variety of sources (e.g., Bourne 1970) suggest that such mortality as occurs from anaesthesia in the dental surgery results in some measure from mishaps at the hands of anaesthetists. Having regard to the greater number of anaesthetic procedures carried out by dentists, the involvement of anaesthetists in fatal cases seems disproportionately large. While this is explicable in part by the inherently greater safety of sedation as compared with general anaesthesia (Chapter 10, page 141), the matter certainly deserves further examination.

Analysis of causes of such deaths is difficult on account of their rarity, and of the sparseness of information usually available, but certain features stand out. Most fatalities seem to fall into one of two types. In one, death seems to be clearly related to some pre-existing disease; the anaesthetist's responsibilities in this field are considered shortly. In the other, the story is that there has been a circulatory collapse or arrest, that despite measures which are apparently efficacious in restoration of circulation there is fatal brain damage. It is necessary to consider possible reasons for this.

Deliberate induction of hypoxia is a thing of the past, with anaesthetists at least. Proficiency in management of airway problems is such that circulatory collapse should not result from obstruction to breathing. In some cases indeed an endotracheal tube has been in use and there has been no suggestion of airway obstruction. Surgical shock of sufficient degree to precipitate circulatory failure is almost unknown in 'office' dental procedures. One is increasingly forced to conclude, with J. G. Bourne (Bourne 1957, 1973) that the damage is due to the fact that the patient is not horizontal, that the elevated position of the head in the dental chair results in failure of cerebral perfusion from an episode of circulatory depression which would otherwise have been easily reversible.

Terminology is crucial here—one should avoid loosely using the term 'supine' because it is not sufficiently precise. It means 'face up', from which it comes to be applied to a reclining or leaning back position. A position in the dental chair which is described as 'supine 160 degrees', or as '70 degrees from the vertical' represents a position in which the patient's head and shoulders are elevated by 20 degrees from the horizontal (Fig. 44). It will be evident to the anaesthetist that the occurrence of circulatory collapse in a patient who is postured thus must be potentially damaging to the brain. Circulatory collapse of any sort should be rare, but such is its lethal potential if the patient's head is elevated, that no position for dental anaesthesia or sedation other than horizontal or head down can generally be countenanced (Love, 1971) (see Fig. 44, page 125).

The patient's health

A serious source of trouble is the overlooking of significant ill-health in a patient whose general appearance does not suggest it. Careful scrutiny of the patient's health is vital, this cannot be done effectively by the anaesthetist asking questions in the course of a brief pre-anaesthetic examination. The eliciting of a history can be time consuming, the return from dental patients in terms of positive findings is small. A questionnaire about general health should be applied to all patients even before booking them for general anaes-thesia—the screening procedure set out in Chapter 6 (page 74) will help to ensure that medical assessment in preparation for general anaesthesia is efficacious and a serious potential source of trouble will not be overlooked. This may not, however, entirely solve the anaes-thetist's problem.

His belief that, if he refuses general anaesthesia, there is no alter-native left but unsupplemented local analgesia, may tend to make the anaesthetist proceed in cases where there is a degree of risk. He is apt to feel 'cornered', to feel that he is being subjected to undesirable pressures. Because of this, anaesthetists who lack a knowledge of dental sedation sometimes suggest rather curious alternatives. The suggestion is frequently put forward that medical assessment should be performed fully and thoroughly at a time well in advance of the planned procedure. Quite apart from the unrewarding nature of this practice noted in Chapter 6 (page 72) the anaesthetist overlooks the fact that, if he refuses general anaesthesia, this still leaves the dentist and his patient in the same quandary whether the notice be long or short. He may suggest that the case be done in hospital—but that the patient still be subjected to the risk of general anaesthesia. Some anaesthetists, recognizing the fact that the dentists find dentistry, particularly restorative dentistry, difficult to organize in hospital have taken the trouble to obtain and equip special premises where general anaesthesia and dentistry can both be performed under near ideal conditions (Keep 1972). They remain blind to the fact that this fails in some measure as a safe solution to the patient's problem—it may really do no more than to protect the anaesthetist's reputation against the possible stigma of a 'death in the chair'.

The vital need is for the anaesthetist to broaden his view and to recognize that there are, between general anaesthesia and unsupplemented local analgesia, satisfactory alternatives which are inherently safer than general anaesthesia. When sedation is carefully applied, in conjunction with local analgesia skilfully given as required, the result is frequently much more satisfactory all round than is the use of general anaesthesia. It would be reasonable for the anaesthetist who has advised against general anaesthesia to administer sedation on the first occasion for this particular patient, this could be regarded as a 'trial'. If the procedure is satisfactory the sedation could very likely be performed by the dentist on other occasions for the same patient.

One envisages co-operation of this type between anaesthetist and dentist in the dental surgery as forming a basis for an ideal pattern of relief of pain and anxiety in dentistry, and the concept will be examined in more detail to point up its advantages. At the same time one will stress those factors which are felt to constitute significant limitations on the safety of sedation when it is given by the dentist without the 'backing' of an anaesthetist.

FUTURE REQUIREMENTS

There is an undoubted need for dentists to be able to supplement local analgesia with some form of safe sedation when this is required.

This can be feasible only if the dentist, on most occasions, works alone—that is to say without the assistance of an anaesthetist whether doctor or another dentist. Practice of this type involves the dentist in 'total patient care', to suit him for this he may well need in the future an education rather broader than the one which he generally receives today. The principal limitation in the dentist of today is lack of knowledge and experience of clinical medicine, and this is a lack of which the profession and its teachers need to take cognizance in many spheres. There are moves towards the concept of total patient care on the part of many dentists which can not be realized fully without radical changes.

In the field of clinical diagnosis of head and neck conditions, without a wider background of clinical diagnosis of pain and of clinical neurology, the dentist can hardly hope to become a diagnostician of any calibre. In anaesthesia, the dental field lends itself to the pursuit of technical skills, but provides a dearth of experience in problems of circulatory and respiratory systems, with the exception of upper airway obstruction. Likewise in oral surgery, the rarity of serious complications in the way of haemorrhage or infection militates against development of clinical excellence: the oral surgeon needs practice in other fields if he is to be well rounded. These deficiencies in the training of the dentist cannot be made good by any teaching, whether at undergraduate or graduate level, in the Dental School: there will be a need to seek closer liaison with the Medical School, and to ensure that graduate dentists are given actual clinical responsibilities in the general hospital if they are to learn adequately the requisite skills.

One recognizes that these views will not find ready acceptance—indeed that they will meet, in many quarters, with bitter disagreement. Dental School teachers in medicine and anaesthesia believe, in general, that they give their students a good grounding in clinical medicine, and tacitly assume that in the course of dealing with patients their knowledge of and capability at diagnosis will steadily develop. In the case of the average practising dentist this hope is generally not realized. In the field of dental anaesthesia there has been propagated for many years the belief that the dentist will manage anaesthesia well if he avoids the 'problem' patient: such a case may be referred to by some catch phrase as 'the brewer's drayman type'. The implication is that the dentist is equipped by his training and subsequent experience to 'recognize the sick patient', and this belief is shared by many practitioners. A fairly long and close acquaintance with practising dentists leads one to have reservations about their clinical capability in this field. A little thought makes plain the reason for this deficiency—they do not practise medicine. Even if the dentist takes a history, it is not supplemented by a clinical examination of the whole patient nor followed by a serious attempt to formulate a diagnosis and then to confirm this by investigation and by consultation at need. Mere contact with patients does not develop skills in clinical medicine: this sounds ridiculously obvious when said, but is undoubtedly a tacit assumption too often made by anaesthetists associated with the Dental School. It needs to be said loud and clear if Dental Anaesthesia is ever to be made soundly based.

A short term solution

How then is the dentist, with these limitations, able to practise sedation safely? One may take as an example the practice in anaesthesia of the oral surgeon on the North American Continent, which is of a very high standard, yet still has limitations. As part of his training, the American oral surgeon may make a detailed study of anaesthesia and gain practical skill in a wide range of techniques in the anaesthetic department of a general hospital, even if his later practice is based on the American tradition in which a nurse or technician administers the anaesthetic under supervision of the surgeon.

A report of some fatalities which occurred in ambulatory patients undergoing anaesthesia at the hands of the oral surgeons in 1965 is instructive (American Society of Oral Surgeons 1966). In several cases it appears that the oral surgeon was aware of the existence of some cardiovascular or other disability in his patient, yet proceeded with anaesthesia. The reason is quite evidently that the oral surgeon would find it impracticable, and generally unnecessary, to refer elsewhere—to hospital for example—every patient in whom some slight defect of general health is revealed. His pressing problem is the accurate assessment of the significance of ill-health shown up by questioning patients.

Proliferation of questions and tests which constitute the surgical 'work-up' of the patient may be expected to achieve little if anything in increasing safety. Consultation with the patient's own physician has a limited value here, for as noted earlier (Chapter 9, page 131) any pre-anaesthetic assessment must be tentative and subject to revision on the basis of patient response to drugs and to surgery. In the case of the patient whose health is not good, one feels that safety may be achieved most readily by consultation with an anaesthetist who is well versed in clinical medicine and familiar with methods of dental sedation. Such a person should be able to conduct anaesthesia or sedation in such a manner as to avert most troubles, and should be able to deal effectively with any problems which may arise. Mere technical excellence in the field of anaesthesia is not enough when patients are to be dealt with who are not healthy. There is no adequate substitute here for the physician anaesthetist in whom there is an integration of clinical medicine and anaesthetic techniques.

In regard to administration of sedation by dentists, certain conclusions seem to be inescapable. Dentists should gain, by practical instruction, a degree of skill in resuscitation and airway maintenance far in excess of anything that they are likely to need. One holds the view, however, that it is also desirable that they confine their practice of sedation to the simplest and safest techniques, and that they be ready to seek the advice and help of a medically qualified anaesthetist—not only for any patient whose health is in doubt, but also for those cases where any but the simplest methods of sedation are to be employed. The immediate and urgent need, therefore, is that medical anaesthetists should receive, as a part of the preparation for their post-graduate qualification, an adequate and realistic grounding in dental anaesthesia and sedation. Teaching, training and talk directed to other objectives will inevitably be largely fruitless in terms of effective contribution to safety.

Modes of practice

The private practice of the average dentist is conducted largely in isolation from his professional colleagues. In these circumstances he is advised to use, as his main form of sedation, low dose nitrous oxide. In selecting an apparatus for administration of this, his first thought should be for safety. Consideration should also be given, however, to the question of use of the apparatus by an anaesthetist for administration of general anaesthesia. An important matter is to decide whether he will use nitrous oxide as such or pre-mixed with oxygen as in 'Entonox' (British Oxygen Corporation). Obviously the separate supply of nitrous oxide and oxygen makes for more flexibility, but the greater inherent safety of pre-mixed gas is important.

Apparatus is available of the 'mix-your-own' type which is extremely safe when adequately maintained. The gas installation can be provided with safeguards by way of non-interchangeable connections and manifold pressure-drop alarms which make it most reliable. Where safety is dependent on mechanical safeguards, however, it is limited by the excellence of primary installation or assembly, and by the quality of the maintenance (Bell 1972). Such services are expensive. The dentist is often a capable technician and may prefer to do his own servicing rather than pay for a tradesman to do what appears to be a very simple job. Only experience can fully teach the pitfalls of an inadequate installation. In the environment of the dental surgery, where apparatus is not subject to the frequent scrutiny of the expert anaesthetist there is much to be said in favour of the very basic safety of pre-mixed nitrous oxide and oxygen (Entonox). Whichever system is chosen it will usually be feasible for the specialist anaesthetist to adapt the machine for general anaesthesia. He needs to be cautious mainly of the 'non-return valve' which prevents rebreathing from the reservoir bag, as this is a feature which is not usual on anaesthetic machines. For the rest, the specialist anaesthetist finds it interesting to use a machine with the built in safety features usual in modern dental apparatus. After experience in the dental office he may tend to look more critically at the safety of hospital anaesthetic machines which mostly lack any safeguard against inadvertent administration of a hypoxic gas mixture.

LESSONS OF DENTAL ANAESTHESIA

The value of dental anaesthesia in teaching has been emphasized already, but it extends beyond mere technical procedures. An enlightened practice of anaesthesia for dentistry provides valuable lessons in management of patients for surgery. Dental surgery is mostly elective and its performance under local analgesia is usually feasible, although this may necessitate several stages instead of one. The high degree of development by dentists of combined techniques of local analgesia and sedation is forcing the anaesthetist to re-think certain problems of management. Surgeons and anaesthetists too readily assume that local and general anaesthesia are alternatives which are mutually exclusive. When a case on a hospital operating 'list' is scheduled for local analgesia, the surgeon will sometimes insist that no sedation or pre-medication be given. Such a decision is usually based on unfortunate experience of patients who have been rendered un-cooperative and irrational by administration of ill-chosen sedation. The anaesthetist, keenly aware of this problem in administration of sedation, may be unwilling to risk upsetting his surgeon for the sake of the patient's comfort.

A change of attitude is overdue. The anaesthetist needs to learn to apply conscious sedation correctly and effectively. The surgeon will do well to cultivate the arts of gentle patient handling and fully adequate local analgesia. With the variety of tranquillizing and sedative agents now available, there is no longer any excuse for the anaesthetist who shirks this responsibility. There is certainly no better field than dentistry in which to learn perfection in selection of agents and dosage, and patient management.

The anaesthetist should go still further. There are patients who need general anaesthesia for their surgery, but in whom supplementary regional analgesia may be of profound benefit. Where a tendon graft to the hand is performed using the foot as a donor site, the fact that a brachial plexus block will not cover the entire procedure does not negate its use. The enlightened hand surgeon will demand that some form of regional block be used to ensure that the patient wakes from his general anaesthetic with a quiescent hand: not restless from pain and making movements which could spell disaster for his tendon graft. There are many fields of surgery in which benefit to the patient can accrue from skilful use of combinations of regional analgesia with sedation or with general anaesthesia. The anaesthetist has a duty to learn these lessons of dental anaesthesia.

The day patient

As a result of increasing demands on hospital beds and escalating costs of in-patient care, increasing attention is being given to the feasibility and safety of performing many kinds of surgery on a 'day stay' basis. Experience of dental out-patient anaesthesia can be of benefit in this area. Three necessary conditions noted for safety in out-patient dental anaesthesia are relevant.

1. The patient must be in good health.

2. The surgery needs to be suitable for out-patient management at the hands of the surgeon who operates.

3. The surgery should be largely free of serious post-operative complications.

The good health of the patient is of paramount importance. Apart from complications related to the surgery, serious problems under general anaesthesia arise principally as a result of pre-existing disease in the patient. The screening of out-patients in regard to their general health must be thoroughly performed, the system described in Chapter 6 (page 73) can form a sound basis for this. The other considerations are surgical, and the anaesthetist should emphasize the need for realistic assessment of the likely course of the surgery and postoperative care.

There is an inevitable tendency to regard out-patient surgery as 'minor' and as such suitable for delegation to a junior. If it is to be feasible and safe out-patient surgery needs at least the scrutiny and oversight of an experienced and capable surgeon. If performance of the surgical procedure itself be delegated, there still should be adequate supervision. Not only is it important to avoid undue prolongation of the surgery, but there may be a need for making quite difficult decisions. There is a need to recognize that a decision for out-patient management is tentative. The possible need for a change of plan, whether it be to abandon the operation or to admit the patient for in-patient care should always be kept in mind. Co-operation between anaesthetist and surgeon is a vital necessity. The idea of the two forming a team is familiar in dental surgery, but it has remained on a rather narrow basis as a rule. From a limited concept of working together in the mouth it needs to expand to a point where the surgeon is able to offer soundly based suggestions about choice of anaesthetic techniques and mode of management—as noted in Chapter 11 (page 152).

Anaesthetic techniques

Out-patient anaesthetic techniques should be simple. The error of trying to achieve simplicity by uniform application of a single method must of course be avoided (Chapter 1, page 7). The correct decision is to choose the simplest technique which is suited to the patient, the surgery and the anaesthetist, provided that a fairly rapid and uneventful recovery can be expected. Sick patients undergoing complex surgery may need complex methods of anaesthesia. Anaesthetists in training see much of these and sometimes need a change. For the anaesthetic registrar who seems to be unduly attached to complexity, a spell in the out-patient dental clinic with an experienced mentor can be salutary. Mention has been made in Part II of just a few of the lessions of practice, of simplicity and of patient assessment which can be so well taught in that environment.

In out-patient anaesthesia a combination of local or regional analgesia with light sedation can be ideal. If the sedative agent used is low dose nitrous oxide, recovery will be almost immediate. The fact that these are simple methods does not mean that they are necessarily easy to learn and apply. The difficulties which the anaesthetist experiences when he attempts this use of nitrous oxide have been dealt with in Chapter 8 (page 110) but it is worth while to master the technique. A vital pre-requisite to any form of sedation is to talk to the patient sufficiently to find out what are his dislikes and worries in relation to the procedure intended. If a patient has a dread of 'the needle' light sedation with some 30 per cent nitrous oxide should be induced even before venepuncture is performed, certainly before injection of local analgesic solution. Because of the repetitive nature of dental treatment, the dentist is well-nigh forced to pander to his patient's wishes in some measure. The anaesthetist should learn by the dentist's example.

Conclusion

It has been said of the specialist anaesthetist who spends his professional life in the administration of general anaesthesia that he is overtrained for his job. The actual administration, it is said, should be performed by a nurse or technician under the supervision of the physician. The latter could thereby cover a greater amount of anaesthesia and be more free for pre-operative assessments, recovery room and intensive care problems. The plan suggested earlier whereby dentist and anaesthetist work together is in some small degree analogous with this, especially when contrasted with the position common in the United States of America, where the oral surgeon supervises the nurse anaesthetist. Should dental sedation develop along the lines suggested, experience gained may well be of value in determining what rôle the specialist anaesthetist of the future should fulfil.

REFERENCES

Chapter 1

AUSTRALIAN DENTAL ASSOCIATION, Victorian Branch (1971) Personal communication.

MINNITT, R.J. & GILLIES, J. (1948a) *Textbook of anaesthetics.* 7th ed., p. 114. Edinburgh, E. and S. Livingstone.

Ibid. (1948b) p. 281.

Chapter 3

BERGSTRÖM H. & BERNSTEIN K. (1968) Psychic reactions after analgesia with nitrous oxide for caesarian section. *Lancet,* **ii,** 541.

BOURNE J.G. (1957) Fainting and cerebral damage. *Lancet,* **ii,** 499.

COPLANS M.P. (1962) An assessment of the safety of the sitting posture and hypoxia in dental anaesthesia. *Brit. Dent. J.* **113,** 15.

COPLANS M.P. & BARTON P.R. (1964) Nasal breathing and the dental pack. *Brit. Dent. J.* **116,** 209.

ENDERBY G.E.H. (1972) Gas exhaust valve. *Anaesthesia,* **27,** 334.

GOLDMAN V., CORNWELL W.B. & LETHBRIDGE V.R.E. (1958) Blood pressure under anaesthesia in the sitting position. *Lancet,* **i,** 1367.

KAYE G., ORTON R.H. & RENTON D.G. (1946) *Anaesthetic methods.* Melbourne, Ramsay (Surgical), pp. 323–324 and p. 460.

PARBROOK G.D. (1964) Hypoxia during anaesthesia in the dental chair. *Brit. Dent. J.* **117,** 115.

Chapter 4

CONSTABLE H. (1964) Cause of death in the dental chair. *Brit. Dent. J.* **116,** 115.

Chapter 5

BROCK R.C. (1947) The etiology of the lung abscess. *Guy's Hosp. Rep.* **96,** 141.

DENBOROUGH M.A., FORSTER J.F.A., LOVELL R.R.H., MAPLESTONE P.A. & VILLIERS J.D. (1962) Anaesthetic deaths in a family. *Br. J. Anaesth.* **34,** 395.

GILSTON A. & RESNEKOV L. (1971) *Cardio-respiratory resuscitation.* London, Heinemann Medical Books.

Chapter 6

SPEIRS R.B. (1953) General anaesthesia for dentistry: a hazardous field of practice. *Med. J. Aust.* **ii,** 376.

Chapter 7

BOWMAN W.C., RAND M.J. & WEST G.B. (1968) *Textbook on Pharmacology.* Oxford, Blackwell Scientific Publications, p. 527.

DRUMMOND-JACKSON S.L. (Ed.) (1971a) *Intravenous anaesthesia.* London, Society for the advancement of anaesthesia in dentistry. 5th Ed. p. 51.

DRUMMOND-JACKSON S.L. (1971b) Loc. cit. p. 214.

FOREMAN P. (1972a) in McCarthy, F.M. *Emergencies in dental practice.* 2nd Ed., Philadelphia, Saunders, p. 202.

FOREMAN P. (1972b). Loc. cit. p. 194.

JORGENSEN N.B., BURNS A.E. & GAMBOA G. (1963) A clinical report on premedication from the Oral Surgery Clinic of Loma Linda University School of Dentistry. *J.S. Calif. dent. Ass.* **31**, 7.

KAYE G., ORTON R.H. & RENTON D.G. (1946) *Anaesthetic methods.* Melbourne, Ramsay (Surgical) p. 322.

WISE C.C., ROBINSON J.S., HEATH M.J. & TOMLIN P.J. (1969) Physiological responses to intermittent methohexitone for conservative dentistry. *Brit. med. J.* **2**, 540.

Chapter 8

BERGSTRÖM H. & BERNSTEIN K. (1968) Psychic reactions after analgesia with with nitrous oxide for caesarian section. *Lancet,* **ii**, 541.

BOURNE J.G. (1957) Fainting and cerebral damage. *Lancet,* **ii**, 499.

JORGENSEN N.B. & HAYDEN J. (1972) *Sedation, local and general anaesthesia in dentistry.* 2nd Ed., Philadelphia, Lea and Febiger, p. 21.

Lancet (1973) Editorial: Hypertension and cerebral blood flow. **i**, 526.

LANGA H. (1968a) *Relative analgesia in dental practice—inhalation analgesia with nitrous oxide.* Philadelphia, Saunders, p. 46.

LANGA H. (1968b) Loc. cit. p. 163.

PERSSON P.A. (1951) Nitrous oxide hypalgesia in man. Copenhagen, Munksgaard. *Acta odont. scand.* **9**, Supplementum 7.

STEINBERG H. & SUMMERFIELD A. (1957) Influence of a depressant drug on acquisition in rote learning. *Quart. J. exp. Psychol.* **9**, 139.

Chapter 9

JORGENSEN N.B. & HAYDEN J. (1972) *Sedation, local and general anaesthesia in dentistry.* 2nd Ed., Philadelphia, Lea and Febiger, p. 28.

PEARLMAN C.A., SHARPLESS S.K. & JARVIK M.E. (1961) Retrograde amnesia produced by anaesthetic and convulsant agents. *J. comp. physiol. Psychol.* **54**, 109.

Chapter 10

BOURNE J.G. (1970) Deaths with dental anaesthetics. *Lancet,* **i**, 525.

BOURNE J.G. (1957) Fainting and cerebral damage. *Lancet,* **ii**, 499.

BOURNE J.G. (1973) Deaths associated with dental anaesthetics. *Lancet,* **i**, 35.

DRUMMOND-JACKSON S.L. (1962) A milestone in intravenous anaesthesia. *Brit. Dent. J.* **113**, 404.

DRUMMOND-JACKSON S.L. (1971a) *Intravenous anaesthesia.* London, Society for the advancement of anaesthesia in dentistry. p. 280, p. 49.

DRUMMOND-JACKSON S.L. (1971b) Ibid., p. 209.

FOREMAN P. (1972) in McCarthy F.M. *Emergencies in dental practice.* 2nd Ed., Philadelphia, Saunders p. 198.

McCARTHY F.M. (1972) Loc. cit. pp. 147, 207.

Chapter 12

AMERICAN SOCIETY OF ORAL SURGEONS (1966) Anaesthesia for the ambulatory patient. 48th annual meeting—pre-meeting conference. Editor N. Trieger, p. 53.

BELL J.M. (1972) Anaesthetic apparatus. *Aust. Dent. J.* **17,** 241.

BOURNE J.G. (1957) Fainting and cerebral damage. *Lancet,* **ii,** 499.

BOURNE J.G. (1970) Deaths with dental anaesthetics. *Anaesthesia,* **25,** 473.

BOURNE J.G. (1973) Deaths associated with dental anaesthetics. *Lancet,* **i,** 35.

GALLEY A. (1974) Quoted in Notes and News. *Brit. Med. J.* **1,** 2 Feb. p. 207.

KEEP V. (1972) A new approach to dental anaesthesia. *Med. J. Aust.* **2,** 1120.

LOVE S.H.S. (1971) In Hunter A.R. & Bush G.H. *General Anaesthesia for Dental Surgery.* Altrincham Sherratt. p. 118 et seq.

TRIEGER N. & CARR S. (1972) In McCarthy F.M. *Emergencies in Dental Practice.* 2nd Ed., Philadelphia, Saunders, p. 164.

INDEX